# *Holistic*
# LIVING

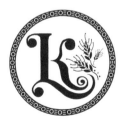

# ADVANCE PRAISE

'*Holistic Living* is a must read for any woman. Kate makes understanding the body (especially hormones) easy and most importantly she provides the actions we all should take to reach our optimal health. With so much information being thrown at us, it's so refreshing to have all we need to know in one place and feel confident that we're making positive decisions with our nutrition and lifestyle.' – **Carla and Emma Papas (The Merrymaker Sisters)**

'Hormone health and ditching diet and fitness fads is the (refreshing!) future of wellness. Kate is on the cutting edge of this, walking her talk.' – **Sarah Wilson, author of *I Quit Sugar***

'This book is so easy to read, full of home truths and simple steps to help you adjust your approach to nutrition and training in order to get your gut and hormones on track, manage stress, improve fertility and ultimately, embrace your femininity. I loved it from the very first chapter!' – **Libby Babet, fitness professional and founder of Agoga and BFU Girls**

'Kate has poured her wealth of knowledge and expertise into this book focusing on hormone health. Her 'easy to understand' approach and explanation allows for many ah-ha moments!' – **Alison Morgan, Health & Wellness Business Coach, www.relauncher.com.au**

'Kate takes a truly holistic and evidence-based approach to helping women eat, move, and live in a way that supports their healthiest hormones... Instead of claiming to know the "perfect" diet and exercise plan we should all follow for optimal health, Kate recognizes that there are many different ways to eat that can all support a woman's health and there is no one-size-fits-all plan...' – **Laura Schoenfeld, MPH, RD, http://www.ancestralizeme.com**

'This book is for any woman who wants to optimise their health...Kate provides solid scientific information that is threaded with personal experience, adding in humour that anyone who has read her first book has come to expect. Kate keeps it real with her recommendations, and the take home messages in each chapter are practical and realistic ... ' – **Mikki Williden, PhD Registered Nutritionist, www.mikkiwilliden.com**

'In *Holistic Living* Kate Callaghan offers a clear, easy to follow guide to wellness for women... It's an amazing resource for all women wanting to look and feel better, but particularly to those facing issues with conceiving, weight loss/gain, fatigue and general hormone imbalance (even or especially to those women having these problems that already consider themselves "healthy")... I love this book and will be recommending it to all of my friends and followers.' – **Claire Deeks, Real food advocate and blogger at www.domskitchen.co.nz**

# *Holistic*
# LIVING

Eat well, train smart and be kind to your body

## KATE CALLAGHAN

For my daughter, Olivia – I wish you abundant health, happiness and love.

**Holistic Living: Eat Well, train smart and be kind to your body**

First published in 2016 in Australia and New Zealand by Finch Publishing Pty Limited. Re printed 2022.

ISBN:
978-0-6454179-0-6 (paperback)
978-0-6454179-1-3 (ebook)

Edited by Jenny Scepanovic
Editorial assistance by Megan English
Text typeset by Jo Hunt
Cover design by Jo Hunt
Kate's Legacy logo designed by Annabell Howie

The image on page 68 is reproduced with permission from the Autism Coach at www.autism.com and the image on page 75 is reproduced from www.cheo.om.ca.

**Medical disclaimer**
This book is not intended as a substitute for professional medical advice, diagnosis or treatment. Always seek the advice of your physician or other qualified health care provider with any questions you may have regarding a medical condition or treatment and before undertaking a new health care regimen.

# CONTENTS

Just in case no-one told you yet ...

Good morning.

You're beautiful.

I love you.

Nice butt.

# INTRODUCTION

Hi, gorgeous! I want to take a moment to thank you for picking up this book. You can go ahead and give yourself a completely non-patronising pat on the back for wanting to find a healthier, more vibrant version of you.

But before we start, let's get something straight. If you're looking for a quick-fix way to get washboard abs and a thigh gap, please put this book down. Now head outside and give yourself a good talking to. You will realise that what you actually need to learn is how to optimise your hormones and get them working for you (rather than against you), so you can be happy, healthy, energetic and sexy (in all senses of the word) for a long, long time. Which will lead you right back to this book! My, oh my! What a coincidence!

In this book you'll discover that whatever your particular goal might be – losing body fat, gaining muscle, reducing bloating, sleeping better, getting more energy or just stopping worrying about what you're eating – you will need to understand your hormones and get control over them. Your hormones control pretty much everything in your body and brain – from how you look (including your ability to maintain a healthy weight), to how you feel, to how easily you fall pregnant. They can even play a role in whether you cruise or struggle through menopause. Hormones are *the* thing. And you need to keep them happy if you want to be happy!

# WHY I WROTE THIS BOOK

Hormone issues have reached epidemic levels. I'm talking things like:

- Polycystic ovarian syndrome (PCOS)
- Hypothalamic amenorrhea (loss of periods)
- Infertility
- Hypothyroidism
- Adrenal issues
- Endometriosis
- Troublesome menopause
- Acne
- Weight issues.

And that's just a start!

Seriously, every single female I see in my practice has messed-up hormones, mostly as a consequence of their own making. This might be a hard pill to swallow, but the exciting thing is that if **you** caused the issue, in most circumstances **you** also have the power to fix it (rather than relying on someone, or something, to fix it for you).

The types of lifestyle issues that I see disrupting hormonal flow include:

- Poor diet – and by this I don't just mean eating dodgy, fandangled foods. I am also referring to those of you who are not eating enough. And this includes those of you who need to lose weight – yes, you might need to eat more to lose weight. Exciting, right? I'm also referring to those of you who eat with a negative mindset. (Feel guilty after that tiny piece of cake, hmmm?) As a result, our gut health is suffering and, as you will learn in Chapter 4 Happy gut = happy hormones, the state of our gut is hugely important in keeping hormones happy. So important that I have written a whole chapter on it. You're excited about this, aren't you?

🌿 Inappropriate exercise – too little or too much can both be problematic for the lady hormones.

🌿 Being an absolute stress-worshipper – in fact, I would have to say that stress is quite possibly the number one contributor to hormone imbalance. Sort it out, chick!

🌿 Letting your inner mean girl take over. I've got news for you: if you aren't willing to show your body a little lovin', don't expect it to show you any lovin' back.

I speak from experience. I have been deep, deep down in the rabbit hole of hormone imbalance. In fact, mine weren't just out of balance, they were pretty much non-existent.

At the tender age of 27 I had the 'ideal body': very low body fat (stupidly low, in fact), six-pack abs ... I was a little ball of muscle. I had always been quite athletic, so this had become my norm.

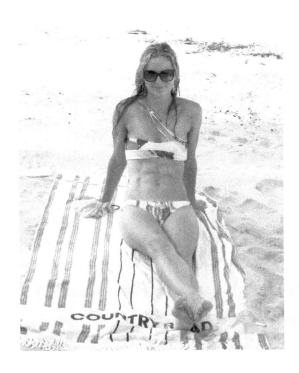

But what was happening on the outside was very different to what was happening on the inside. I was infertile, my bones were breaking down, my thyroid was sluggish, I had no energy as my adrenals were burnt out, my sex drive was a thing of the past, and my recovery from exercise was less than stellar. So while I might have looked healthy, I was actually far from it.

Why? I was diagnosed with hypothalamic amenorrhea. In layperson's terms, this basically meant my brain had stopped communicating to my ovaries to produce a healthy menstrual cycle and ovulation. It had received the message that reproduction was best avoided with this little lady. All of this was a result of the following, self-inflicted, factors:

- Inadequate energy availability – I'm talking food. I was exercising too much (2–3 hours a day) and eating too few kilojoules, and too few carbs, to compensate.
- Too much psychological stress.
- Insufficient body fat.
- Taking the oral contraceptive pill, which I did for over ten years!

As a result of beating my body into submission, I was told by many experts that I wouldn't be able to fall pregnant without fertility treatment.

Here's the thing. I'm stubborn. Stubborn as a mule. So when someone says to me, 'You can't'. I say, 'Watch me!' And so began my journey into healing hormones.

The solution to my problem? Eat more, exercise less, put on some body fat and get stress levels under control. Of course, this was easier said than done. I had my crazy female brain telling me that I should look a certain way in order to be accepted by society, which is where the whole self-love thing came into it. I talk about this in Chapter 8: Be kind. (Please don't skip this part, it's super-important.)

I am happy to report that after applying some simple and mostly free, (other than the food, but you gotta eat, don't you?) strategies that you will learn about in this book, my period returned, my fertility was restored, and at the time of writing this book, I have a healthy eight-month-old daughter who was 100 per cent naturally conceived. Take *that* fertility experts!

Unfortunately, I see many women making similar mistakes and suffering the consequences. Lady hormone problems aren't really talked about that much. If you have an issue, the response is usually, 'We have a pill for that.' My mission is to spread the word that there are other ways to heal your body. If you want to take the drugs, go for it, but know that in most cases, there are other, more natural, and probably longer-lasting, options. And if you *do* choose to take the drugs, doing so in combination with the food and lifestyle strategies you will find throughout this book will no doubt improve the results.

So this is why you won't find anything about how to get washboard abs, a thigh gap, or how to lose some ridiculous amount of weight in a short amount of time. These aesthetic traits that we perceive to be so important do not necessarily mean we are healthy. In fact, they can be quite damaging. I've been there. And it's not fun. Instead, I hope that women around the world, both young and old, can learn from my mistakes. Treat your body with warmth and respect. Nourish it well with good food and movement, as well as kind, loving thoughts and words.

# MY HOLISTIC LIVING PHILOSOPHY

I am a nutrition nerd. This nerdiness has kept me kicking on in the health and fitness industry for over fifteen years. I'm what they (the elusive 'they') call a 'slashie': dietitian/nutritionist/personal trainer/group fitness instructor/former beauty publicist/mother/lover of all things fermented (I'll expand on this one in Chapter 4: Happy gut = happy hormones). Two degrees, multiple certifications and several years of self-induced stress later, I have found that my passion is helping others to become holistically well.

I advocate an ancestral healing approach. Sounds pretty airy-fairy, doesn't it? My philosophy is all about holistic living, which is not about just what you eat, but also the way you move your body, how well and where you sleep, what stressors you are faced with and how you manage (or mismanage) them, the products you use on your body and around your home, and what you enjoy doing during your downtime (if you have any). On top of this, emotions and beliefs are explored to provide a well-rounded picture of the *whole* person.

The ancestral approach to healing involves taking all of these factors into account and seeing how they impact the various systems of your body (such as the digestive system, adrenal glands, skin, brain, thyroid gland and reproductive systems), and how you can make improvements through subtle, non-medical shifts by balancing your hormones.

In a nutshell (because I expand on all of this later, but I know you want to suss out what my caper is before you spend money on this book – you're still standing in the book store, aren't you?), my philosophy looks a little like this:

Eat well.

Train smart.

Be kind.

## Eat well

***When diet is wrong, medicine is of no use. When diet is correct, medicine is of no need.***
– Ayurvedic proverb

Food has the power to nourish, heal and energise our bodies. As the famous Greek doctor Hippocrates stated 'Let food be thy medicine, and medicine be thy food.' Over the last century, this innate wisdom has been lost among the advancements in food science, medicine, technology and an ever-growing 'I'm too busy' mentality.

As a society, we are no longer truly nourishing ourselves with food. Instead we are opting for pre-packaged and processed fake foods that cause us more harm than we could have ever imagined. To truly heal ourselves, we need to keep our digestive system healthy (see Chapter 4: Happy hormones), reconnect with real, whole, nutrient-dense foods and eat the way nature intended. This is why I advocate an 'ancestral healing approach' (see Chapter 1: An ancestral approach). Chapter 5: Eat well gives you the details. In the meantime, here are my four simple food guidelines:

- If you can grow it, pick it, hunt it; if it will rot; if it was once alive (plants included) – eat it.
- If it is processed, don't eat it.
- Food should always be enjoyed – 'healthy' does not have to mean 'tasteless'.
- Create an awareness and appreciation of how you eat and where the food you eat comes from.
- Choose quality over quantity.

## Train smart

The conventional 'kilojoules in, kilojoules out' recommendations for weight management have created a society of sick, over-trained, injured, tired and bored individuals. Seeing exercise as a way to burn off that extra slice of cake or glass of bubbles you had on the weekend is not going to create the healthy body you want. In fact, it's incredibly unhealthy and damaging to your overall wellness. Exercise is a form of stress on the body, which means a little can be of huge benefit to your wellbeing, but too much is just as detrimental as none at all. My key exercise principles are:

- Train smarter, not longer, doing a variety of exercises and movements that you enjoy.
- Never view exercise as punishment for something else.
- Always allow adequate time for rest, recovery and regeneration.

See Chapter 6: Train smart for more on putting the fun back into exercise.

# Be kind

Stress, negativity, lack of sleep and lack of play can undo all of the benefits we obtain from eating well and training smart. It's true. See Chapter 8: Be kind to find out why. It's time to start being kind to yourself (and others) *now*.

- ❧ Try to get seven to eight hours of sleep each night so as your body can adequately rejuvenate.
- ❧ Incorporate stress management into each and every day. (Chapter 7: Manage Stress is loaded with fun ideas to keep you chilled out.)
- ❧ Play! Do something fun with friends or family on a regular basis that is unrelated to work or exercise.

# WHAT YOU'LL FIND IN THIS BOOK

What *won't* you find in this book? Seriously, when you're all about the holistic healing biz, you need to cover everything, which is why I wanted to create a bit of a hormonal bible for you. A place you can turn to when you're lost in a hormonal deluge, searching for answers and just a little overwhelmed and confused about all the different opinions out there. So here's what this book has in store for you.

**Chapter 1: An ancestral approach** gives you an overview of healing your hormones – the whats, the whys and the hows. You'll see how a holistic, ancestral approach to healing incorporates nourishing all the systems of your body simultaneously: eating whole, nutritious foods we were designed to consume; exercising in a way that's fun, invigorating and biologically appropriate; and keeping your stress levels in check. This, my friends, is how to get your hormones in their happy place, so you can experience more energy, better sleep, better skin and a better sex life. (Yes!) Using an ancestral approach to healing is how I managed to restore my own hormonal balance, it's the basis of how I get my clients out of hormonal havoc, and it's how you, too, can find yourself in hormonal bliss.

**In the next two chapters**, we get a little sciencey on all things hormones – what they are, how they work, and what it looks like when things are out of whack. Don't be turned off by the whole science aspect of it. Yes, it does get a bit nerdy, but I break things down for you (and include some handy visuals) to help you understand what is going on with your body, which means you then have the power to decipher what your body is telling you, and how to go about fixing it. Knowledge is power, and all that.

A healthy gut and liver are essential when it comes to happy hormones. Why? Well, your gut is where you will absorb all of the nutrition from the food you eat. When your gut is in good shape and you're getting all of the nourishment from your food, your hormones (and every cell throughout your body) will be kept in tip-top working order. Your gut is also vital for eliminating used-up hormones, and making sure that they don't get reabsorbed into your body. If you're not pooping properly (we'll troubleshoot this one, too), this can lead to hormone imbalances.

Then we have your liver, which is responsible for detoxification (getting rid of waste products such as old hormones and toxins from your environment). You know this, right? But do you know how to ensure you are detoxifying properly? In **Chapter 4: Happy gut = Happy hormones**, I explain how to show your liver some lovin' on a regular basis to help keep your hormones happy. Hint: it doesn't involve any sort of juice/water/lemon or maple syrup cleanse.

**Chapter 5: Eat well** – the title says it all. If you're not eating nutrient-dense foods that provide an abundance of vitamins, minerals, antioxidants, fibre, carbs, fats and proteins (all the good stuff!), then your hormones are going to be all over the place. In this chapter, I give you the lowdown on everything you need to know about what you put in your pie-hole – what to eat, what not to eat, and how much to eat. And, of course, how these factors help your body achieve perfect hormonal balance. I even give you a delightful nutrient-filled, delicious meal plan to get you started on your nutrient-seeking path to hormonal bliss.

Exercise is such an important part of maintaining a healthy body and mind, but are you overdoing it? Or perhaps you're under-doing it? Are you using it as punishment rather than pleasure? **Chapter 6: Train smart** tells you all about how to move in ways that are going to rejuvenate rather than deteriorate your body, while also helping you to achieve your wellness goals without jeopardising your hormonal health.

Stress! I know it's not the sexiest of topics, but it's a huge factor in hormonal balance. In fact, it's often the main contributor to hormonal unhappiness I see in my clients. In **Chapter 7: Manage stress** I explain how stress causes hormonal woes and give you lots of ways, ... (not just 'You really should meditate') to help manage it.

**Chapter 8: Be kind** is all about being kind to yourself. I know, it sounds like the stuff of crunchy hippies, but believe me, it's an integral part of your holistic journey to achieving a healthy lifestyle and happy hormones. When you're kind to yourself, as well as others, you realise your self-worth. You realise that you are worthy of respect, and of being treated well. When you realise these things, you are more likely to engage in all of the other wonderful strategies suggested throughout this book like (eating and moving well, and keeping stress low), and less likely to beat yourself up – physically, mentally or emotionally. This can be a bit of a sticking point for many of us ladies, but once you push through, I promise you will be so much happier and healthier that it will radiate from within!

And, of course, it would be criminal of me not to include some recipes so that you can get started on cooking yourself some hormone-lovin' foods. Turn to **Chapter 9: Recipes** to find yourself a bunch of wholesome, nutrient-rich recipes that will not only nourish your hormones and help you get your glow on from the inside out, but also taste amazing. Promise.

# WHO NEEDS THIS BOOK?

Are you a woman? Yes? Then you need this book. (Actually, as a side note, I reckon some men could do with reading it too, just so they can understand us a little better, don't you think?) But in all seriousness, I wrote this book for women like me – those who have found themselves up the proverbial hormone creek without a paddle after years of over-training and under-eating, or perhaps just being an absolute stress-head.

I wrote this book for the women who might have been following a paleo-style diet, which is working great for Joe-next-door, but seems to be taking things in a less-than-desirable direction for them. (We'll chat more in **Chapter 5: Eat well** about why the conventional low-carb paleo diet is not such a great idea for most women).

I wrote it for the women who have been told that they would be unable to fall pregnant naturally and would need fertility treatment, with no alternatives offered.

I wrote it for the women who need to lose weight and are advised to 'just eat less and exercise more', even though they have been doing that to no avail for the past umpteen years.

I wrote it for the women who are sick and tired of being told that their hormones-gone-bad symptoms are 'just-a-fact-of-being-a-lady-and-accept-it-or-take-a-pill'.

If you would like to look better, feel better, and bounce through each and every day with vigour and vitality, then this book is for you.

# YOU HAVE THE POWER TO HEAL YOUR HORMONES

You can heal your hormones, and keep them balanced long term, through simple strategies and tweaks to your food, exercise and stress management, as well as by showing yourself a little love each and every day. And this book gives you a big ol' bunch of these strategies that you can implement right away! Hurrah!

Here are some ideas to get you started.

- Optimal wellness is so much more than simply eating good food, but food is an excellent starting point.
- You can't out-train a bad diet.
- Even if something is common (e.g. fatigue, lack of menstruation, painful periods, joint pain, sugar cravings, 3 pm energy slump), that does not mean it is normal. It just means that there are heaps of other women just like you with messed-up hormones.
- Just because your parents had it, doesn't mean you will. We can manipulate our genes through diet and lifestyle choices (this all belongs to a field called 'epigenetics', which is way too complex to delve into in this book). Just know that factors such as what you eat, how you move, where you live and what you think have the ability to turn on and off certain genes, making you more or less susceptible to certain health conditions. So if you're one of those women saying, 'Oh well, it's in my genes to have X condition' and just accept it as part of your fate, I call BS. You are responsible for how things turn out.
- You deserve more. Stop simply surviving and start thriving!

The power for change, for healing and for happiness is in your hands. Literally, if you're holding this book! As they say, knowledge is power. I want to educate you. Inspire you. Give you that little nudge in the butt that you need to say, 'Hell, yeah! I am fabulous, I am in control, and I love and respect myself enough to treat myself like the queen that I am.' And I mean this in the most non-arrogant way.

Whatever you do, never allow another person to be your health guru and dictate exactly how you should live and what you should eat. If someone tells you that they know everything there is to know about nutrition, and they know what the perfect diet is for all humans, run the other way and don't look back. Nutritional science is in its infancy – there is still so much we are yet to discover. What we know now is just the tip of the iceberg. Not only this, but no-one knows what is best for you more than you do yourself – you are your own guru.

We are going to be forever learning about nutrition and what is best for us. But we do know that by getting back to basics (with food, exercise and mindset) by learning from what our ancestors (who were relatively free of the chronic diseases and hormone imbalances we are faced with today) valued and how they lived their lives, we can give our bodies the best possible chance. Let's lay the foundations for healthy, happy hormones, build upon it as and when it works for us.

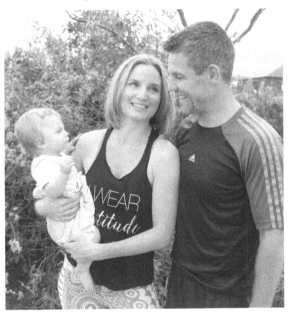

So that's what this book is for – providing you with the what, the why and the how of addressing the root causes of your hormonal imbalances through diet and lifestyle strategies. Holistic healing is not about quick-fixes. It's about long-term, sustainable change.

Remember, good things take time, so be patient with yourself and enjoy the journey.

Kate xx

# AN ANCESTRAL APPROACH

*If civilised man is to survive, he must incorporate the fundamentals of primitive nutritional wisdom into his modern lifestyle.*
– Dr Weston A Price

It's no secret that many aspects of modern society are messing with our hormones. Food is increasingly devoid of the nutrients required to serve as the building blocks and engines of our hormones. It is also being pumped full of dodgy ingredients, such as sugar, vegetable oils and ingredients you can't even pronounce, which contribute to a whole cascade of inflammation and hormonal hell (you'll read about this in Chapter 5: Eat well).

We are also moving in ways that are biologically inappropriate for us as humans. We're either doing too much, which is placing a stress on the body and depleting sex hormones; doing too little (sitting is the new smoking, haven't you heard?); or forcing our bodies into cutting some shapes that just aren't right. (Chapter 6: Train smart is your go-to on this topic.)

On top of this, we have a crazy amount of psychological stress (hello, Chapter 7: Manage stress). This stress depletes our sex hormones and leaves us feeling crummy. And finally, we are exposed to an exorbitant amount of environmental toxins that mess with our hormone balance, which is why they are often referred to as 'endocrine disruptors' (endocrine = science-speak for hormones).

Taking an ancestral approach means paring things back. Right back. In all aspects of life – food, movement, mindset, environment. It doesn't mean hiding away in a cave and gorging on a wildebeest that you just hunted down. (I suspect this is the image that you might have when I mention the term paleo but I'll explain my take on this soon.)

In this chapter, you'll learn about the aspects of ancestral living that we can adapt to our modern world, to nourish our bodies, help our hormones flourish, and keep us glowing like a glitter-bug for many years to come.

## MY TAKE ON PALEO

Many of you have probably heard of a paleo diet. Generally, people will be somewhere on a spectrum of attitudes towards such an approach to eating. There are the paleo diehards (I was there once), who believe that paleo is a lifestyle not a diet (I do agree with this) and is the one and only way to live, with no room for leeway (I disagree with this).

Then at the other end of the extreme, we have the paleo-is-a-fad cohort, who believe just that – the paleo diet is a passing craze, or worse, it is dangerous to one's health. I disagree with this when such a way of eating and living is implemented with a little common sense.

However, I do understand where these paleo-is-a-fad people are coming from. Paleo has become a little bit faddy and is surrounded by quite a bit of negativity. Some of these more trendy, hard-core versions of paleo are best avoided, especially by females, as they can be quite restrictive in a number of ways (carbs!) that can harm our hormones (you'll learn more about how later on and in Chapter 5: Eat well).

So let's, for a moment, forget about what the media portrays as paleo and have a look from a healthier perspective.

I like to think we can sit somewhere in the middle of the two extremes by using a paleo (or what I prefer to call 'ancestral') template to build on and suit our own individual tastes, preferences and requirements.

Taking an ancestral (or evolutionary) approach to something means looking at how our ancestors lived – the way they ate, and moved, and how they interacted, promoting optimal health and happiness through hormonal balance, and then adapting these practices to suit our modern lifestyles. It involves looking into how we evolved and asking questions about the potential harmful aspects of our modern lifestyles that have deviated from that of our ancestors.

The paleo diet gets its name from the era it refers to, the Paleolithic Era, which ended around 10 000 years ago. The diet involves emulating how our ancestors of this era lived. While this is a very romantic idea, I don't think we need to go back quite this far to learn some valuable lessons about how to live. We could simply look back to how our grandparents or great grandparents lived. In fact, many people are now talking about something called the 'mid-Victorian diet' (around the 1800s – not too long ago, really), which shows that living as our more recent ancestors did is a potentially wonderful way to avoid unhappy hormones and the chronic diseases of modernity.

Even more recently than this, in the 1930s, a super-inquisitive dentist named Weston A Price (who I quoted at the start of this chapter) headed out on some epic adventures to visit fourteen traditional cultures around the world, studying the way they lived and the foods they ate, and how they lacked the chronic diseases that plague modern society. He's often referred to as 'the Charles Darwin of nutrition'.

What Dr Price was actually looking for was causes of dental decay and oral deformation, and he found that this provided a window to a person's overall health, as these issues were often the result of nutrient deficiencies. (And remember, nutrient deficiencies are a sure-fire route to hormones going haywire, which I talk about in Chapter 5: Eat well).

Places Dr Price visited included isolated villages in Switzerland, Gaelic communities in the Outer Hebrides, Eskimos and Indians of North America, Melanesian and Polynesian South Sea Islanders, African tribes, Australian Aboriginal peoples, New Zealand Maori and the Indians of South America.

What the members of all of these societies had in common were beautiful straight teeth, freedom from decay, resistance to disease, emotional stability, strong, healthy bodies and, you guessed it, the happiest of hormones. And I quote from the Weston A Price foundation:

*'When Dr Price analysed the foods used by isolated primitive peoples, he found that in comparison to the American diet of his day, they provided at least four times the calcium and other minerals, and at least ten times the fat-soluble vitamins from animal foods such as butter, fish eggs, shellfish and organ meats.'*

Superb! Just superb! You're going to see in Chapter 5: Eat well why these traditional super-foods are so wonderful for nourishing your hormones and promoting optimal health and wellness. If you're interested in learning more about Dr Price's research, I can highly recommend his book ***Nutrition and Physical Degeneration***.

This is why I prefer the term ancestral over paleo, because we can learn a little somethin' from pretty much ALL of our ancestors, not just the ones who hung out in caves. (But I'll probably still drop the whole paleo term here and there, so don't hold me to it.)

# LIVING LIKE OUR ANCESTORS

So how did our ancestors live? What made their diet and lifestyle so health-promoting? And what did they avoid that is ravaging our hormones today? Most importantly, what aspects can we take on board to help keep our hormones happy? The key, really, is getting back to basics and acknowledging the things in life that really matter.

## Nourishing with whole, unadulterated food

To be honest, we don't (and probably can't) know exactly what all traditional societies ate. However, what we do know is that our ancestors ate fresh food or they fermented fresh food, which improved in nutritional value over time. Believe it or not, they didn't have Tim Tams back then. The food they ate was of the highest quality – no chemicals, no added hormones, and no factory farming.

They ate foods that were nutrient-dense. By that I mean foods that were jam-packed full of goodness (vitamins, minerals and antioxidants). And they opted for foods that were produced locally, in a sustainable manner, and were most likely organic (fertilisers and pesticides are a relatively recent invention).

Just like today there is no one-size-fits-all diet, back then there was no one single ancestral or paleo diet – food choices would have varied depending on geographic location and time of year. For example, we understand that the Inuit subsisted mainly on whale meat and blubber, which meant that their diet was incredibly high in fat; whereas the Kitavans of Papua New Guinea indulged in a diet high in carbohydrates, obtained from roots and tubers. Then we have the Masaai, who still today feast on milk, blood and meat from the cattle that they raise themselves. (Of course, there were some fruits and veggies gathered by the communities tossed in there, too.)

What did all of these communities have in common? They were all at one with nature. And they all experienced excellent health, free of many of the issues caused by inflammation and messed-up hormones that we suffer from today, such as diabetes, obesity and autoimmune conditions.

What was similar in all traditional diets was what was absent: packaged and processed foods, refined oils and carbohydrates, artificial flavours and colours, preservatives, genetically modified organisms, factory-farmed and hormone-laden animals and foods devoid of nutrients due to soil depletion.

Generally, when speaking of a paleo or ancestral diet, the following food groups are excluded (we'll go into more detail in Chapter 5: Eat well about why, and whether or not this exclusion is 100 per cent necessary for everyone).

- Processed foods – think crackers, biscuits, donuts, chips, fruit juice, modern soy foods, instant soups, canned foods, soft drink, ice-cream, lollies.
- Grains – wheat, oats, rye, barley and the like.
- Legumes – beans, lentils, chickpeas, you get the gist.
- Dairy – milk, yoghurt, cheese.
- Plus the other usual culprits such as sugar, artificial sweeteners, preservatives, flavours, colours and refined oils.

Flick to Chapter 5: Eat well to learn all about how you can apply these food principles to your life.

## Getting moving

The common school of thought is that we need to 'eat less and exercise more' or 'if some exercise is good, more must be better.'

We exercise as a means to an end – to lose weight, to get a six-pack or a thigh gap, to burn off excess kilojoules, to give us energy that we don't have (as a result of going too hard for too long), because it is something we think we **should** be doing.

(By the way, stop saying 'should' right now! Turn it around and say 'I could, but [fill in your reason for why you aren't doing X here].')

This is not how our ancestors would have moved. They would have walked. A lot! How often do you walk? Most people I know will drive to work, sit down all day, then drive to the gym and do an hour of exercise, expecting everything to be merry. Unfortunately, this is not how our bodies were designed to move.

Our ancestors would have sprinted occasionally, for example, when they were hunting, or running from a wild beast. That's right – occasional and intermittent intense activity.

Our ancestors would have lifted heavy things from time to time. You can still see examples of traditional societies engaging in this type of activity if you head over to Africa and visit the Maasai, where you will notice the women (yes, the women) lifting heavy objects such as piles of wood and buckets of water on a regular basis. That's right, ladies – it's important that you are physically strong and resilient. Put away the bright pink 2 kilogram dumbbells right now and go and pick up something worthwhile.

When they sat down, our ancestors would do so on the ground, or in a deep squat position, as opposed to in a chair, which is probably doing more harm than good, especially for the kiddies, in my opinion.

If your hormones are out of whack, exercise can make or break you. You'll learn more about how to exercise appropriately to help heal your specific hormonal issues in Chapter 6: Train smart.

## Enjoying social interaction with loved ones and the wider community

We are so stupidly busy these days that no-one has time, or at least no-one makes the time, to spend with friends and family. Peeps back in the day would have enjoyed regular social interaction with members of their family, their friends and others located nearby. Admittedly, this was a touch easier for them as they didn't have 9-to-5 jobs (or other extended hours away from the home environment), nor did they have to commute to and from work, or pick up the kids from school, or do a massive pile of washing, or vacuum the house and clean the bathroom. Phew! Don't you wish you could travel back in time?

So while life might not be like it was back then, making it a little more difficult to catch up with friends and family, this doesn't mean we shouldn't prioritise it. Spending time with loved ones has a calming effect on your central nervous system, getting you into 'rest, digest and reproduce' mode where your hormones are at their happiest.

## Incorporating daily stress management

Let me tell you now: no matter how spot on you are with healthy eating and regular exercise, if your stress levels are through the roof, then chances are you are going to struggle to get your hormones in balance.

While I can't really tell you if our ancestors sat on a rock and meditated every day, what I can tell you is that all of the other factors, such as catching up with friends and family, and not having a million things jammed into their smartphone calendar, would have helped keep their stress hormones in check and, therefore, other hormones in balance.

Back then, release of stress hormones would have been intermittent, not chronic as they tend to be today. For example, if you were being chased by a tiger, you would certainly expect that your stress hormones, particularly adrenaline, would be released. Why? Because they would crank up your heart rate, increase your breathing rate and divert blood flow to your muscles, which would enable you to run like the wind and, hopefully, escape said tiger. Then once the prospect of imminent death had passed, and you had a chance to compose yourself and brag to your friends that you managed to out-run a tiger, those stress hormones would return to baseline and you could return to your natural state of 'rest, digest and reproduce'.

Now, stress hormones are chronically elevated as we are faced with more stressors (though, admittedly, not as stressful as the jaws of a tiger), and faced with them more often. Also, dare I say it, most of us tend to overreact to these stressors. Have a think about it. How often do you find yourself sitting in traffic, working yourself up about all the things you need to do at home, and how rude that driver who cut in front of you was, and OMG there are so many red lights! Arghh! The world is against me and nothing is going right! Before you know it, you're shaking, your heart and breathing rate have increased, and you're just sitting in your car. There is no tiger. And has all of this effort changed the traffic situation? Didn't think so ...

All of this unnecessary stress is depleting your much-needed sex hormones. The ones that keep you radiant, energetic and not feel like you're going to bite someone's head off. In Chapters 7: Manage stress and 8: Be kind, you'll find some easy-to-implement strategies for mitigating the negative effects of stress and self-destructive behaviours while keeping your hormones content.

## Obtaining adequate, restful sleep

Ahh sleep. Blissful sleep. So, so important to our overall health. Like stress, if your sleep is inadequate, then all other attempts at hormonal balance will be thrown out the window. Seriously, just one night of dodgy sleep can increase your insulin resistance, and your tendency towards hormone issues such as diabetes, PCOS and obesity. Not to mention the cravings for sweet stuff you'll feel the next day!

Our ancestors would have slept when it was dark and woke with the light (or something close to it). Their circadian rhythms would have been spot on. Why? Well, I guess because they had no other choice – they didn't have electric lighting, they didn't have smartphones or computers, non of the things that keep us up at night with their blue light telling our brain to stay awake. The only light that our descendants would have been exposed to at night would be the occasional campfire, which they would sit around singing **Kumbayah** and toasting marshmallows on sticks (well, maybe not this last part). As you know, the light that fire gives off is orange, not blue. Orange light doesn't suppress the release of melatonin, our sleep hormone, like blue light does. Blue light also triggers cortisol – your waking-up and your stress hormone!

# Embracing realistic and fertile bodies

As depicted in art, ancestral women's natural curves were revered, as opposed to trying to become smaller and smaller. It is likely that, to them, what we do to our bodies today (and why) would seem laughable. There was no 'thinspiration' or 'thigh gap' or #strongisthenewskinny. Even now, if you travel to Africa and talk to women about diets, they will think you're crazy. Trust me, I've been there. They told me I was too skinny. And they were right.

The ancestral woman was healthy. Her body was how it was – she did not try to force it into some perceived 'ideal' mould. She was often curvy and had fat stores in all the right places (boobs, booty and yes, thighs), which symbolised fertility. She was sexy. She chose the most nutrient-dense foods to nourish her body, and even chose special foods during the pre-conception period, which were known for their hormone and fertility-boosting properties. She respected her menstrual cycle. She did not run around at 100 miles an hour trying to be perfect at every little thing. She did not compete with other females around her. We could learn a thing or two from her. And you will, in Chapter 8: Be kind (an absolute must-read chapter!).

At the same time, the ancestral woman did not face issues with obesity. The foods she ate, and the way she lived her life, allowed for perfect hormone harmony. Healthy weight maintenance was effortless. She didn't even have to rely on counting kilojoules and checking the scales each and every day. Shock horror!

As a woman, adopting an ancestral lifestyle means respecting and listening to your body, and responding to its needs with kindness, patience and love … always!

# DISPELLING SOME MYTHS ABOUT THE PALEO DIET

It's great that paleo/ancestral lifestyles are getting more attention; however, unfortunately, they are still being portrayed as a carnivore's feast, where animal protein has to form the majority of all your meals. Indeed, when you mention paleo to many people, they will often say:

- 'Urgh! It's just too much meat!'
- 'It's not sustainable, or environmentally friendly.'

Let me clarify that paleo is not, nor should it be, a meat-centric diet. Ideally, it should be a plant-based diet with adequate fats and proteins sprinkled on top. In Chapter 5: Eat well we'll take a look at what your plate should be made up of.

And here some other untruths about the paleo diet:

- **Paleo is low in fibre.** If we were to just eat meat and meat alone then yes, we probably would be lacking in poop-bulking, bacteria-feeding, hormone-regulating fibre. (Nice image in your head right now, isn't there?) However, most ancestral diets around the world were crazy-high in fibre – much higher than our dietary guidelines recommend today. Some studies suggest levels were up around 150 g per day. (Contrast this with the measly 30 g recommendation we have today.) That's a poop-load of fibre, pun intended! So, when planned appropriately, you should be getting more fibre than what is typically recommended.
- **Paleo is low-carb.** This one is controversial. Many people say low-carb is best. Many people say low-carb is bad. I'm of the opinion that everybody is different and should adjust their carbohydrate (and fat and protein) intake accordingly. I have seen some people excel on a low-carb diet, while others fall flat on their face. This whole carb thing is pretty important, and it is often a sticking point for many people. There tends to be quite a bit of carb-phobia around. Carbs are not scary. We'll see later on why females should include some carby-goodness in their diets to keep their hormones happy.
- **Paleo is dairy free.** Strictly speaking, yes paleo is dairy free. However, some people who follow this way of eating find that they do just fine, and even thrive, on dairy,

especially unprocessed, full-fat milk. The Masaai of Africa continue to flourish on fresh milk (and blood, and meat). Who are we to say then, that they shouldn't have any dairy, if they are feeling like a pig in mud?

🌿 **You need to eat a block of butter each day.** Paleo is not Atkins. While butter is incredibly delicious and nutritious, there is no need to go overboard.

🌿 **Paleo is expensive.** Pfft! You know what is expensive? Cancer is expensive. Heart disease is expensive. Diabetes is expensive. A nutrient-dense diet that could prevent or even reverse these diseases? Not expensive, relatively speaking, and a whole lot less painful. Eating a paleo diet does not mean that you have to dine on organic eye fillet, oysters and caviar! Head to Chapter 5: Eat well to see how to feed yourself well without breaking the bank.

🌿 **Paleo is unsustainable.** If we all relied on grain-fed, factory-farmed cattle then yes, the world would probably implode (not necessarily factual). However, paleo diet proponents nearly always emphasise grass-fed, humanely raised animal produce. See Chapter 5: Eat well for more details on grass versus grain-fed livestock.

🌿 **Paleo is lacking in nutrients.** Again, pffft! That is what I have to say to that! Cast your eyes to the meals at the back of the book. There are a tonne of veggies there, providing plenty of vitamins and minerals. And that's just the start. We add eggs, liver, bone broth, sauerkraut, kombucha, beet kvass, kefir, meat, chicken, fish, nuts, seeds, yoghurt, avocado, coconut, berries, bananas, olive oil. Please, tell me, what nutrients is this diet lacking in?

🌿 **Paleo man died young, so we will also die young if we follow this diet.** If we look a little more closely, we can see that the reason for the low life expectancy was due to things like infection from wounds or broken bones. Paleo men were not lucky enough to have the medical treatments for acute injuries that we have today. They also had to face things like freezing cold nights without central heating, and being chased by carnivorous animals. So the data, in this sense, is a little skewed.

To the naysayers out there, I have this to say. Just for a moment, take your ego out of it, forget about the guidelines that the government has told us to live by, and ask yourself, 'Does this make sense?' Why not try it and see? You might be pleasantly surprised!

# COMMON MISTAKES MADE BY WOMEN 'GOING PALEO'

Most of the information put out onto the inter-webs surrounding an ancestral lifestyle is written by males, the majority of studies cited are based on males, and pretty much all of the images put out promoting what a paleo diet can do for you involve half-naked men with very little body fat and bulging muscles.

If you put two and two together, you realise that this information is *for* males, and perhaps needs a slight tweak to suit us sheilas.

However, we often tend to grab information and run with it, quite literally. Then we end up in quite the predicament with hormones gone awry, feeling pretty shabby and not getting the results we had hoped for.

Unfortunately, advice pertaining to women who are interested in following an ancestral approach to food, exercise and lifestyle is lacking (albeit growing now). Being the emotional creatures that we are, it is not surprising that we latch on to promises of fast weight loss, six-pack abs and abundant energy, despite being presented with an image of a buff *male* body.

Remember, ladies, we are not designed to be this lean – we are designed to have a little junk in our trunk, and boobs up top. They are sexy. They are a sign of fertility, health and abundance. Embrace them instead of constantly trying to change them. I must add, though, if you are naturally skinny and lacking in the boob department, this is not to say you aren't sexy – sexiness, I believe, comes from what's on the inside, rather than the outside. Getting a little deep now ...

The following are probably the most common mistakes I see women making when going paleo.

## Not eating enough carbohydrates

We'll go into this in more detail in Chapter 5: Eat well but in a nutshell, lack of carbs can mess with your adrenal, thyroid **and** sex hormones, leaving you in a very underwhelmed, dodgy skin, no-sex drive, infertile state. Inviting?

What do I mean by low-carb? Well, this is different for everyone, but as a general rule, I would say less than 100 g of carbohydrates per day would classify as a low-carb diet. So what does 100 g actually look like on a plate?

- 1 banana
- 1 apple
- 1 cup sweet potato
- 1 cup parsnip

= 89 g of carbohydrates.

I would put money down that some of you are looking at this amount and thinking, 'Holy moly that looks like a lot of carbs', which probably means you are batting way below your requirements. Am I right or am I right?

## Low-carb diet plus HIIT

HIIT is an acronym for high-intensity interval training – you work really hard for a burst of time, cranking your heart rate up, followed by a period of rest, allowing your heart rate to come back down. Then you do it again. And again. And perhaps again.

So many women come to me in a hormonal heap who are following a low-carb, paleo-style diet while simultaneously doing CrossFit, F45 or other high-intensity exercise five times a week. I'm sorry, but this will not actually get your hormones in optimal shape to lose body fat; it might even increase it! Head to Chapter 6: Train smart for more ideas on keeping your exercise in a hormone-friendly zone.

HIIT is a very effective style of training if you are clever about it and team it with the right nutrition, and perform it when your body is feeling up to it. However, one thing you need to be aware of is that HIIT is what we call glycolytically demanding, which means it uses glucose (aka sugar, aka carbs) as fuel. This style of training helps to burn fat after the fact but during the workout, sugar is what your body likes to gobble up. It is simple science, friends.

So, if you do not fuel your body with sufficient carbs, what's a body supposed to do? Now, the low-carb purists will tell you that you don't need carbs as your body can make it from proteins (a process called gluconeogenesis), or by breaking down glycogen, stored glucose (termed glycogenolysis). This is correct. However, to do this, your body will need to release cortisol, which, as you will learn about in the next two chapters, is your number one stress hormone. Cranking up cortisol on a regular basis is going to strain your adrenal glands and deplete your sex hormones. Which = bad (a little word math for you there). This is something called the pregnenalone steal (stay tuned for more details in Chapter 7: Manage stress).

Also note that your stores of glucose are located in your liver and muscles. Once your liver stores are used up, your muscles will be broken down for fuel. Now isn't that a little counter-productive? Do you really want to be doing all that hard work, only to have *less* muscle and proportionately more fat?! No, you don't. Having an appropriate amount of lean tissue is essential for healthy hormonal metabolism. And having some body fat is equally important for ensuring your hormones are in optimal condition. Say what? Yep! In Chapter 6: Train smart you'll learn why a little booty is essential.

Not only that, but when cortisol ramps up and pulls glucose into the blood, insulin needs to pull rank to shuttle that glucose back into your cells to be used as fuel or to be stored as fat. Often, women who train like this will notice that they have some stubborn belly fat that will not shift, no matter how much they train. That's cortisol saying, 'Hey there! I'm just going to hang out here until you fuel your body right.' This can be avoided by incorporating a little smart carbage into your diet.

I'll let you in on a secret – I have been firmly in the low-carb camp in the past. I went through quite an extended period of time eating a high-fat diet, with only 10 per cent of my kilojoules coming from carbs. I was also eating inadequate kilojoules (around 5880 kilojoules or 1400 calories per day) while doing a *lot* of exercise. As in *every day* I would do some sort of intense exercise. No rest for the stupid wicked, right?

In grams, 10 per cent of kilojoules coming from carbs on my previous, insufficient diet was around 35 grams. That's a little over a cup of sweet potato. In a whole day! Ridiculous! My body was starving, in more ways than one. No wonder my sex and thyroid hormones went into hibernation! In Chapter 5: Eat well we will delve into what an appropriate amount of carbs might be for you and your goals.

# Intermittent fasting

Intermittent fasting (IF) involves going for an extended period of time (usually sixteen hours) without food, while keeping your food intake to the remaining time window of eight hours. It's another way of mimicking the whole paleo lifestyle of famines followed by feasts (as there would not have been the constant food availability that we have today).

There are many benefits that can be obtained from IF, such as:

- Improved fat burning and weight loss.
- Decreased insulin levels.
- Increased cellular repair.
- Reduced oxidative stress and inflammation throughout the body.
- Improvements in heart disease risk factors, such as blood pressure, cholesterol and triglycerides.
- Prevention of cancer (although studies have thus far only been done on animals).
- Improvement in brain health and possibly prevention of Alzheimer's disease (again, more human research is needed here).

That all sounds super, doesn't it? It does. And it is! However, much of the research has been conducted on males, not females like you.

In my practice, I see IF causing more health issues than health improvements in the ladies. Often, clients will come to me after doing IF for a while and complain of things such as trouble sleeping, regular anxiety and irregular periods – all symptoms of a hormone imbalance disaster!

Why is this? Often, with IF comes kilojoule restriction, and when you are consuming inadequate kilojoules, as we will discuss later in Chapter 5, your body gets the message that you don't have the supplies required for reproduction. Thus, sex hormone production is down-regulated, leading to menstrual, fertility, sleep and mood issues. Boo!

Men, those lucky buggers, aren't quite as susceptible to this hormone fallout as they aren't the ones doing the baking of the baby in the oven. From an evolutionary perspective, if you are essentially starving yourself on a regular basis, pregnancy will be perceived as a very hazardous business as risk of death (maternal and foetal), will be more likely due to the huge amount of stress that growing and nourishing a mini-human places on your body.

So, word to the wise – be very careful when toying with intermittent fasting. If you're adamant that you want to give it a go, do so when you are not stressed (you've mastered all the strategies in Chapter 7: Manage stress), when you're sleeping well, and your periods are regular and healthy. Also, try to eat the same kilojoules as you would in a normal day, but compress the 'feeding window' into a shorter time period rather than eating a significantly less amount of food. And keep an eye on things. If you notice your periods become lighter and/or less regular, if you stop ovulating, if you develop skin issues, if you can't sleep, or if you're becoming moody, maybe give it a rest. Don't be stubborn. It's not a competition.

## Under-eating

This is the common approach to losing weight and a mistake made by many women, not just those following a paleo-style way of eating. In fact, women who haven't decreased their kilojoules in an effort to lose weight over the years (whether needed or not), would probably be in the minority. After all, we have been told for many years now that in order to lose weight we must eat less and exercise more. In fact, I was taught at university that if someone was eating less than they were burning off and not losing weight, then they must be lying. How arrogant is that?

If you're in this camp of not losing weight, despite starving and sweating yourself silly at the gym on a daily basis while feeling like a failure, I want you to stop right there. Chin up, beautiful. You are not a failure. You have been failed by the advice that has been provided to you.

Unfortunately, while you can trick your body in the short term by restricting kilojoules and burning off fat, after a while it will cotton on to what you're doing. It will sense that you're in a famine and start to hold on to every little morsel of food that you put into your mouth, regardless of how many aerobics classes you punish yourself with. Not only this, but your hormones are getting messed up in the process.

Again, this comes back to how things were back in the time of our ancestors. If we indeed were in a famine, our brains would sense this, slowing down our metabolism (by down-regulating thyroid hormones – see Chapters 2: Hormones working well and 3: Hormones going haywire for more) and storing anything we consume as fat. This was an especially efficient process in females. After all, the survival of our species is dependent on our fertility and our ability to carry a mini-human. And if there is insufficient energy around, baby-making ain't gonna happen, friends.

We'll chat more about kilojoules, how many you might need to have healthy hormones and achieve optimal wellness (as well as weight loss and maintenance), and how too few can mess you up, in Chapter 5: Eat well.

All of these elements provide a nice, holistically nourishing baseline to help keep our hormones happy. See it as a starting point for where to head with your diet and lifestyle.

Is this the perfect lifestyle for you? Maybe, maybe not. There generally is no one perfect diet. (And on that note, let's get rid of the idea of perfection right now.) We are all different and so have different needs, and these needs may also change throughout your life. What works for you now may not work for you in ten or even five years' time. If you want optimal health, you need to learn to listen to your body. If something isn't working for you, then change it!

I wish it were as simple as saying, 'Eat exactly like this and all of your problems will be solved.' Life unfortunately does not work like that. So, let's start with this ancestral template. Let's then tune in to what our body is telling us, and tweak things appropriately. Sound good? Good!

## Recap time

- ❧ We can learn a lot from our ancestors about keeping our hormones happy: eat good food, move in ways that are biologically appropriate, keep stress levels in check, spend time with loved ones, and be kind to yourself.
- ❧ There are many myths surrounding paleo/ancestral diets, including that they are meat-centric, low in fibre, expensive and unsustainable.
- ❧ To keep your hormones in a state of bliss, avoid the common going-paleo mistakes like cutting out all carbs, training to excess (with inadequate fuel), intermittent fasting (unless applied in a smart and realistic manner), and under-eating in general.
- ❧ There is no one, perfect diet. Use ancestral principles as a starting point, then experiment and find out what works for you, your hormones, and your happiness.

Now ... time to learn all about these hormones we've been talking about. Get your nerd caps on, don't be scared, it's really interesting and not too technical.

# HORMONES WORKING WELL

*Every day, think as you wake up, today I am fortunate to be alive,*
*I have a precious human life, I am not going to waste it.*
– Dalai Lama

Ready to learn all about your hormones and how they affect how you look, feel, think and act? Buckle yourself in for some science fun – and no that is not an oxymoron!

Hormones are chemicals produced by our body that are released into the blood or lymphatic system, and act like messengers telling specific organs what to do. We produce numerous hormones, and each has its own exclusive target organ that will respond to its messenger in a characteristic way. For example adrenaline, which is produced by the adrenal glands, will tell the heart and lungs to increase their rate of activity so you can escape the hypothetical grizzly bear that is chasing you.

These messengers are made in our endocrine glands, which are best demonstrated pictorially, don't you think? Check out the illustration on the next page.

All of these glands, and the hormones they secrete, will be of relevance to you and your health (other than the testis, obviously!), and the function of all of these little babies can be affected by what you eat and how you live your life. So let's get on top of those things to ensure you're in tip-top shape, hey?

# Major endocrine glands

**Male   Female**

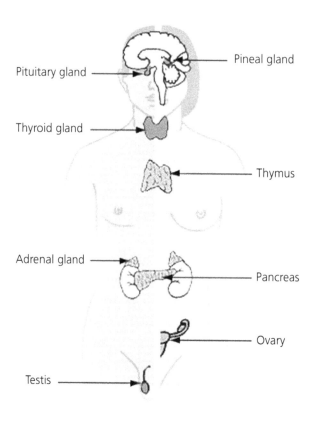

Pituitary gland

Pineal gland

Thyroid gland

Thymus

Adrenal gland

Pancreas

Ovary

Testis

In case you were wondering, hormones play a key role in a range of functions important for the ladies, including:

- Menstruation
- Fertility
- Menopause
- Immune health
- Bone health
- Heart health
- Weight management
- Mood
- Skin health
- Blood sugar regulation.

Hormones get blamed for a lot of things (most notably our tendency to be a little crazy sometimes), but they are essential to our very being and, when in balance, they can make us feel pretty fantastic! When our hormones are humming along as they should be, we can expect to experience the following:

- Abundant energy throughout the day (without the 3 pm slump when you will take a bite out of anything, including that slightly annoying co-worker who you can usually tolerate).
- Stable moods.
- No food cravings.
- Glossy hair and clear skin – hey, sexy lady!
- Easy weight maintenance.
- Healthy sex drive.
- Good sleep quality.
- Regular menstrual cycle.

❧ Smooth transition into menopause and post-menopause. (Yes, you read that correctly; menopause doesn't have to be the scary disease that it is made out to be, it should be a bit of a non-event, really.)

Sounds good, right? How many of those can you happily check off? How many seem completely elusive to you? Now's the time to do a quick self-check. How do you feel right now? How many of the above happy hormone benefits do you experience? Write them down. Go on …

Right. Now, let's backtrack a little bit and talk about some key hormones for female health and vitality, and why they are important.

# IT ALL STARTS IN THE BRAIN …

If you were to look deep into your brain, you would find a little pea-sized structure called the *hypothalamus*. Let's call it H (as it is your master control centre, and I'm a lazy typist sometimes).

The role of the Master H is to maintain homeostasis in the body, which is basically a fancy term for balance, or stability. Master H is like the traffic control centre, receiving and responding to information about your body's temperature, hunger, blood pressure, blood glucose, heart rate, stress, metabolism and more. If things are out of whack, it is the role of Master H to get on the job and return things back to their sweet spot. It does this by communicating to a nearby gland, called the *pituitary gland*, to release hormones, which will then communicate to particular endocrine glands throughout the body (refer to previous illustration on page 34) to either up the ante, or chill out a little with their hormone production.

The key hormones released by Master H that I will focus on (there are others) are:

- **Corticotropin-releasing hormone (CRH)** – sends a message to the pituitary to get the adrenal glands kicking into gear, releasing corticosteroids such as cortisol (your stress-management system).
- **Gonadotopin-releasing hormone (GnRH)** – tells the pituitary to release follicle stimulating hormone (FSH) and luteinising hormone (LH) to help the ovaries produce sex hormones and regulate the menstrual cycle and ovulation.
- **Oxytocin** – your love hormone. Oxytocin is involved in orgasm, sleep cycles, the ability to trust, bonding and the release of breast milk. This feel-good chemical is also released through hugging and touch, which we will chat about later.
- **Thyrotropin-releasing hormone (TRH)** – tells the pituitary to release thyroid stimulating hormone (TSH) to give the thyroid gland a nudge.

Note to self: Master H is needy. We must look after it if all else is to run smoothly. I talk about this more in Chapter 7: Manage stress where I discuss the HPA axis (hypothalamic-pituitary-adrenal axis. (Say that five times fast!)

# HORMONES PRODUCED THROUGHOUT THE BODY

The hormones I have listed on the next several pages are just *some* of those produced by your body's endocrine glands. These are the ones I see most often contributing to optimal health (or lack thereof) in the women that I chat with on a daily basis. When these are in balance, you can expect to look and feel *a.mah.zing* each and every day because, as you will learn, they are not just involved in fertility and menstruation, which is often the misconception when one thinks about hormones.

Oh, and one more thing that you really should know. Most of the hormones discussed are produced from, wait for it, cholesterol! Yes, that big bad substance that everyone demonises, suggesting that, when it comes to cholesterol, 'the lower the better'. Let me tell you now, and please imprint this firmly in your brain: without cholesterol you don't have a lot of the hormones oestrogen, progesterone, testosterone or cortisol – they all need it! Got it? Good.

# Oestrogen

Oestrogen is perhaps the most well-known female sex hormone. It is produced mainly by the ovaries, but also by the adrenal glands (this is an important factoid to remember!), which sit atop our kidneys. Oestrogen is also produced by your fat cells. (Again, stamp this fact in your brain now and wait for your mind to be blown in Chapter 6: Train Smart – a little body fat is needed for hormone health. Less is *not* better.)

When it comes to the menstrual cycle, oestrogen encourages the maturation of the eggs, as well as the thickening of the lining of the uterus as a way of making a nice, cushy bedding for a potential baby to grow and develop in. During menopause, ovarian production of oestrogen ceases, which results in menstruation also concluding, hence the name 'meno-pause'. Oestrogen is also responsible for the production of fertile cervical mucus.

As well as promoting a healthy, fertile menstrual cycle, oestrogen plays a role in bone health by:

❧ stimulating bone formation.
❧ suppressing bone resorption, whereby bone is broken down and the minerals are released, resulting in a transfer of calcium from bone to blood.
❧ inhibiting osteoclast activity – these bad boys are responsible for breaking down bone.
❧ boosting expression of vitamin D receptors, thereby helping to get vitamin D to do its job in bone building.

Let's have a look at how your lady hormones, oestrogen and progesterone (and a couple of other hormones), dance together over the month to promote a healthy reproductive cycle. Here's what it should look like, in point form for sake of brevity:

❧ A regular healthy cycle is 28–35 days long from the start of one period (this is your day 1) to the start of the next period. In a perfect world, a new menstrual cycle should start every 29.5 days. Guess what else is 29.5 days long? The lunar cycle!

❧ During the first half of your cycle, the follicular phase, oestrogen is dominant, your basal body temperature is relatively low, your follicles are maturing with the help of follicle stimulating hormone (FSH), your uterine lining is thickening, and your cervical mucus is increasing and becoming more fertile.

❧ Around midway through your cycle, ovulation occurs with the help of luteinising hormone (LH) when an egg bursts out of the mature follicle and waits patiently (about 12–24 hours) for a super-star sperm to come along and join forces with it.

❧ You will (generally) only ovulate ONCE per month and are fertile for about three days, if that. (Yet we are advised to take the oral contraceptive pill month-round. Hmmm ...)

❧ During the second half of your cycle, your luteal phase, progesterone increases, your temperature should increase (to create a nice little oven for a potential bun to bake), the mature follicle from which the egg was released will turn into the 'corpus luteum', and your cervical mucus may dry up.

❧ Twelve to sixteen days after ovulation, if you are not pregnant, progesterone levels will fall and you will experience menstruation again as the uterus sheds its lining.

❧ Throughout your menstrual cycle, as your hormones fluctuate, your cervical mucus will change as follows:

  • days 1–5: Menstruation (aka bleeding).
  • days 6–8: Dry, no cervical mucus
  • days 8–12: Increasing cervical mucus; might be white and creamy, like Clag glue (sorry for the visual, but at least you know what to look for).

- days 13–16: Ovulation will bring about fertile mucus, which looks a little like egg white and is quite slippery/stretchy. (Yes, it's okay to touch it; it's not filled with flesh-eating bacteria.)
- days 17–28: Mucus may go back to white and creamy and will gradually become drier towards the end of the month.

A healthy reproductive cycle is vital for *all* women, not just those who are concerned with baby-making. This cycle, and any deviations from it, serves as a little monthly report card. If your menstrual cycle is out of whack, this is your body whispering to you to make some changes in your diet and lifestyle. Be sure to listen to this whisper before it becomes a yell and everything comes crashing down, which I talk about in the next chapter.

Finally, oestrogen is important for heart health. Low levels of oestrogen can adversely affect something called nitric oxide – a chemical produced in our body that helps to regulate the health of our blood vessels. Low levels have been associated with an increased risk of heart disease.

Oh, and you are probably interested in this little point: oestrogen is a big deal when it comes to keeping your skin all smooth and supple, and your locks luscious.

# Progesterone

Progesterone is our other key female sex hormone. It is released during the second half of our menstrual cycle (the luteal phase) by the corpus luteum (this is what the follicle is called after it has released an egg). Progesterone also helps to create a nice warm environment for the implantation of a fertilised egg, and will crank up quite significantly in pregnancy. Think of this one as pro-gestation (gestation meaning pregnancy).

Another not-so-well-known fact about progesterone is that it has an anti-anxiolytic effect, which basically means it helps to mitigate anxiety. If you find that you get anxious, especially the week before your period, you might have low progesterone.

# Testosterone

I know what you're thinking, that's a manmone (man hormone). Correct, it is the dominant sex hormone in males, but we ladyfolk also produce a small amount of testosterone.

Why is testosterone vital for us? For a number of reasons, including:

- bone strength and lean muscle development – important, I'm sure you would concur?
- overall sense of wellbeing and happiness – sounds pretty good!
- sex drive and sexual pleasure – yes, please!

# Cortisol

Cortisol is often portrayed as the bad boy and, indeed, if it gets let out for too long and/or too often, it can cause quite a few issues, which I delve into in the coming chapters.

Cortisol is your main stress hormone, and is produced by your adrenal glands. Along with adrenaline and noradrenaline (aka epinephrine and norepinephrine), your body releases cortisol when it senses danger and/or stress in your life. This helps to move glucose (blood sugar) into the blood to use for fuel, and direct blood flow towards your heart, lungs and muscles in order to help you to fight or flee from the inherent danger, whether perceived or real. At the same time, blood flow is directed away from digestion and reproduction, as these are not required in order to run from the hypothetical tiger that wants to eat you.

Cortisol also plays a role in your sleep–wake cycles (called circadian rhythms). Levels will peak in the morning to help get you bouncing out of bed and then (should) decrease over the day as melatonin increases to make you sleepy at night.

A few other interesting activities cortisol partakes in (along with your other adrenal hormones):

❧ The production of thyroid hormones – specifically the formation of your active thyroid hormone (the one that is needed to do the work).
❧ Decreasing inflammation by reducing the secretion of histamine (think about what you use antihistamine medications for) and helping with the stability and integrity of your cells.
❧ Influencing memory formation.
❧ Controlling electrolyte balance.

## Thyroid hormones

Your thyroid gland is a butterfly-shaped gland in your neck. It uses iodine (and other essential nutrients such as selenium) to produce two key hormones:

❧ **Thyroxine (T4)** – the inactive thyroid hormone.
❧ **Triiodothyronine (T3)** – the active thyroid hormone. (T4 also gets converted to T3 at various places around your body, including your gut and your liver, so long as these organ systems are in tip-top shape).

Your thyroid gland produces these hormones in response to a different hormone that is released by the pituitary gland (in your noggin), called thyroid stimulating hormone (TSH). If you need more thyroid hormone, TSH will increase. If you need less thyroid hormone, TSH will decrease. TSH acts like a thermostat for your body.

But what does your thyroid actually do? Well, everything, really. No kidding. Every single cell in your body relies on thyroid hormones for the regulation of their functioning. Most notably, the thyroid is a metabolism regulator. Too little thyroid hormone and things will slow down (and you may gain weight). Too much and everything will be put on high speed (sounds great in theory, but it's not a nice feeling and not at all good for your health). It's all about finding that Goldilocks sweet spot for your thyroid hormone. You really want to be looking after this one as it can affect, and be affected by, other hormones. They're all interconnected, you see!

## Insulin

Produced by the pancreas, the main role of insulin is to help regulate our blood sugar levels. When our blood sugar levels increase (for example, after eating a carb-filled Tim Tam or experiencing stress), insulin will be released in order to push this sugar (glucose) into the cells where it can be used or stored, as opposed to hanging out in the blood where it can potentially do damage to your blood vessels.

## How female hormones differ from male hormones

Well, to be honest, they don't. We all have the same hormones, and they all have similar actions. The difference lies in the amounts of these hormones that ladies have in contrast to the fellas.

Females have more oestrogen than testosterone, whereas the opposite is true for the boys. However, things can swing the other way for both sexes, with oestrogen increasing for males and testosterone increasing for females. Both of these scenarios are not ideal and can lead to unwanted side effects in both sexes. (Think acne, facial hair and male-patterned baldness in females; and man-boobs, or 'moobs' in males.)

What I have found in my work, and in my research, though, is that the female hormonal system is a little less resilient than men's. The gents seem to be able to deal with less-than-ideal circumstances better than the ladies. If we take an evolutionary perspective, this makes sense …

Imagine if, in a time of great stress (such as a famine), your hormonal system were to keep on truckin' on, with your reproductive system functioning as it should be, and you fell pregnant. This would place your life, and that of your unborn child, in great jeopardy. Pregnancy and breastfeeding are energy-intensive, stressful situations for the female body (trust me, I've been there). If there is a lack of food and/or stress levels are sky-high, chances of survival for both mum and bub are decreased.

I see this all the time in my practice. And I hear it daily from frustrated women.

❧ 'Hubby and I are following the same diet and he has lost so much weight but mine hasn't budged, I have gained some!'
❧ 'My best (male) friend and I have been working out together – he's got an impressive six-pack whereas mine looks more like a beer belly.'
❧ 'The boy down the road has been doing intermittent fasting and says he is feeling (and looking) fab. I tried this and feel like poop!'
❧ 'How come he can get away with [insert dodgy food and lifestyle choice here] whereas if I do this I [insert adverse health effect here].'

Note to self: you are not a male. Your hormones are more sensitive than a man's. So let's celebrate being a *wo-man* and be smart about things, all right?

## Recap time

❧ Hormones are 'messengers' that tell specific organs in your body what to do – the message cascade begins in your brain at the hypothalamus and pituitary and then travels to numerous endocrine glands throughout your body, which then produce hormones to cause a desired effect.
❧ Key hormones that influence women's health are oestrogen, progesterone, testosterone, cortisol, thyroid and insulin.
❧ When these hormones are in balance, you can expect to look, feel and perform like one red-hot mama!
❧ Most of these hormones are made from cholesterol – so eat the yolks!

# HORMONES GOING HAYWIRE

*You're entirely bonkers. But I'll tell you a secret. All the best people are.*
– Lewis Carroll

So now you know that your hormones are important in helping you feel vibrant, sexy and juicy (yes, I said juicy), what does it look like when things are out of whack?

The following are some of the most common hormone-related issues that I see in women.

## LOW, OR NO, SEX DRIVE

Yes, I'm going straight to the pertinent matters in life. If you would rather clean the toilet bowl than have sex with your significant other then alarm bells should be ringing. You might have *low testosterone*, which is responsible for getting you fired up for some between-the-sheets action, or you could have *high cortisol*. Both of these bad boys are produced by your adrenal glands, so employing stress-reduction techniques (see Chapter 7: Manage stress) can help to reignite the spark.

Another cause of low libido could be low oestrogen, which helps with the production of cervical mucus to make lovin' more enjoyable. If your oestrogen is low, one of your key symptoms might be vaginal dryness. And if you have no idea about how moist your nether regions are, (sorry to those who hate the term moist, I know you're shuddering a little right now) it's about time you became acquainted. This small piece of information can tell you a lot about what's going on with your hormones (see page 39 for more on cervical mucus).

Note: If you're taking the oral contraceptive pill, you probably won't notice any cervical mucus as this is one of the ways this drug helps to prevent conception – by drying everything up and making it hard for sperm to swim to their destination. (Loving all of the visuals in this book yet?)

## TRACKING YOUR CYCLE

Grab yourself an app such as Kindara and start tracking your periods and your fertile signs and symptoms (including your cervical mucus), throughout the month, as well as things like headaches, sore breasts and acne. This is a great way to see if your sex hormones need a little boost.

For extra brownie points, why not start tracking your basal body temperature, too? This is a handy (and free and painless) way to get a window into your hormone function, and not just your sex hormones. You can also see how well your thyroid and adrenals are doing. All by putting a little stick under your tongue each morning. Here's how.

- ❧ Buy yourself a digital thermometer.
- ❧ Stick said thermometer under your tongue as soon as you wake up each day (before moving/eating/drinking).
- ❧ Record temperature in Kindara app, which will give you a nice little graph to look back on month after month.

❧ If you wake earlier or later than usual, make a note of this, as this can affect your result.

❧ If you got on the booze the night before or if you are ill, make a note, as this can also affect your result (usually increases the number).

And here are the kind of issues you can pick up.

❧ If you have more than five entries below 36.4 degrees Celsius, your thyroid could need a bit of a pep talk, especially if you notice other signs associated with underactive thyroid function (see page 51 where we talk about constipation and feeling cold).

❧ If your temperatures jump up and down quite significantly throughout the month (they will naturally go up and down a little), your adrenals might be tired.

❧ If you do not notice a bi-phasic pattern, where in the first half of your cycle you have relatively low temperatures then, at around halfway through your cycle, your temps spike up and stay relatively higher for the rest of your cycle, you might not be ovulating.

❧ If your temps do spike in the middle of your cycle but then only stay elevated for ten days or less before coming back down again, you might have something called a 'luteal phase defect', which is marked by low progesterone.

If you are seeing these sorts of things, take your charts (yes, take three or four months' worth) to a health professional. Avoid diagnosing yourself. Step away from Dr Google! All roads end up at cancer with Dr Google. If you're interested in educating yourself more on tracking natural fertility and hormone health signs, check out the works of Francesca Naish and Katie Singer. I cannot recommend these highly enough.

# ACNE ALONG THE JAWLINE OR ON THE BACK (AKA 'BACKNE')

If you have acne, your testosterone might be **too high.** (See how you need to find a nice middle ground?) This can often be a result of insulin being too high, which causes oestrogen to do a little sex-switch into testosterone. These are key signs that you might have something called polycystic ovarian syndrome (PCOS), which is one of the most common hormonal problems faced by women, and is a key player in many cases of infertility.

Some other things to look out for if you suspect you have PCOS include:

- Difficulty losing weight (although slim women can also have PCOS).
- Hair in less-than-desirable places, such as the upper lip, chin, breasts and back.
- Irregular, or absent, periods.
- Unexplained hair loss.
- High blood sugar levels.
- Polycystic ovaries, as shown on an ultrasound scan.

PCOS is a syndrome (a collection of symptoms) and should not be diagnosed solely on having cysts on the ovaries. Other conditions, such as hypothalamic amenorrhea, can also cause polycystic-like ovaries.

# IRREGULAR, OR ABSENT, MENSTRUAL CYCLES

Your monthly lady holiday, or lack thereof, should be seen as the canary in the coalmine. If your cycles are irregular or worse still, absent (amenorrhea), and you're not going through menopause, take this as a strong indicator that your hormones (and general health) need support. Don't leave it too long, or your fertility, bone and heart health may suffer.

There are a number of reasons for menstrual irregularities and amenorrhea, including:

- Elevated stress (high cortisol).
- Excess exercise (again, high cortisol).
- Eating poorly and/or not eating enough
- Low body fat (can contribute to low leptin, which is responsible for telling the brain that there is sufficient energy around for reproduction).
- The oral contraceptive pill.
- PCOS.

If your period is MIA, and you have ruled out PCOS, you will most likely see low oestrogen, progesterone and testosterone on your blood test results.

The most common cause of missed periods that I see is hypothalamic amenorrhea (HA), which I have suffered from. In simple terms, HA basically means your brain (hypothalamus and pituitary) has stopped communicating to your ovaries, as a result of:

- excess psychological stress.
- inadequate energy availability (ie exercising too much and/or eating too little).
- low body fat (although this is not always the case).
- taking the pill.

It is essential to get on top of healing HA as long-term consequences include, but are not limited to, osteoporosis, increased risk of heart disease and infertility. If you think you might have HA, check out my website (www.theholisticnutritionist. com), where I give you loads of information and an e-book on how to heal HA. Many of the strategies in this book are also handy for getting your Aunt Flo to return.

# ANXIETY, INFERTILITY, SPOTTING PRIOR TO YOUR PERIOD AND EPIC PMS

Here, you're probably looking at low progesterone. Progesterone is essential for ovulation (see page 40), and also for maintaining a pregnancy by creating a nice, warm little oven for your developing bun. If it is low, you may struggle to fall pregnant and/or maintain a pregnancy.

Progesterone also has a lovely anti-anxiolytic effect – it decreases anxiety. When it's low, you can expect to feel on edge, especially pre-period. You might also notice some spotting a few days before your period. Oh, and if you find you're a little 'Jekyll and Hyde' when it comes to your periods, your progesterone is probably in the dumps.

# BELLY FAT, LOW IMMUNITY, SLEEP PROBLEMS AND BLOOD SUGAR SWINGS

Hormone issues aren't pretty, are they? These are all warning signs that you're burning the candle at both ends and your adrenal glands are running on empty. You have relied on cortisol, your main stress hormone, for too long and it is shutting up shop and leaving you high and dry.

This high cortisol is also messing with your insulin levels, contributing to blood sugar swings (do you get hangry before meals?), and possibly, further down the line, boosting up testosterone levels. Are you starting to see how everything is interconnected? This is why we need to look at healing our bodies in a holistic way, as opposed to looking at hormones and systems in isolation, as is common practice in many medical communities.

# CONSTIPATION, LOW ENERGY, WEIGHT GAIN, FREEZING HANDS AND FEET

If you're nodding your head right now, you could have a sluggish thyroid. Your thyroid gland controls your metabolism and is your body's temperature controller (see page 42). Some other things you might notice if your thyroid is running on empty include:

- depression
- brain fog
- dry skin
- thinning of the outer thirds of your eyebrows

- thinning hair on your head
- high cholesterol
- low basal body temperatures (see the box on page 46 for how to track this).

# WHAT MAKES HORMONES GO CRAZY?

A number of factors can contribute to hormonal imbalance, including:

- Stress
- Exercise (too much or too little)
- The pill
- Antibiotics and poor gut health
- Poor liver health
- Pregnancy, and all things related to it
- Environmental toxins – think air pollution, cosmetics, skin products and cleaning products, to name a few.

## Is stress throwing off your hormonal balance?

If a gun was held to my head and I had to say what the **one thing** contributing to hormonal imbalance was, I would say it's stress. Here's why stress should be something on your hormone-health radar.

Remember how in Chapter 2: Hormones working well I talked about Master H (the hypothalamus)? Well, it's back. The hypothalamic pituitary adrenal (HPA) axis is an important player when it comes to addressing hormonal imbalance.

Our adrenal glands sit atop our kidneys and have the task of producing many hormones, including those that regulate stress (cortisol, adrenaline, noradrenaline) and blood pressure (aldosterone). They also produce sex hormones (although to a lesser extent than your ovaries).

When all is well, everything is in balance and your stress hormones are under control. However, if, like I used to be, you are a stress-head who lets every little thing get to you, your stress hormones may remain chronically elevated.

This is a problem. Not only does this communicate to your brain that you are in a stressed (fight or flight) state, thereby switching off your rest, digest and reproduce state, it also slows down production of sex hormones by the adrenal glands. This happens via a process known as the pregnenalone steal. I go into more detail on this in Chapter 7: Manage stress.

## I thought exercise was good for you?

It is! But it's all about balance! Just because some is good doesn't mean more is better. On the other hand, a complete lack of exercise is clearly not healthy at all.

Sit tight! Chapter 6: Train smart rummages through all things exercise and hopefully clears things up for you.

## How does the pill cause my health to suffer?

The oral contraceptive pill is an innocent little pill that many of us go on at a young age to make life easier for ourselves: for contraception, to improve skin, or to fix issues such as PCOS and endometriosis. However, the pill does no such thing. It acts as a Band-Aid. Chances are, when you eventually come off the pill, those issues will still be there.

# HOW THE PILL WORKS

The pill delivers hormones that mimic the physiologic activity of oestrogen and progesterone produced naturally by the body. Quite high levels are provided by the pill, which inhibit the release of follicle stimulating hormone (FSH) and luteinising hormone (LH).

FSH is responsible for stimulating the development of follicles in the ovaries, one of which will go on to become the dominant follicle, which has the potential to release an egg that can be fertilised down the road.

LH is predominantly responsible for ovulation and for probing the production of progesterone in the second half of the menstrual cycle, to promote a viable pregnancy.

So that's how it works to prevent pregnancy.

The pill, unfortunately, has many side effects that most of us aren't usually aware of:

- Increased risk of cardiovascular diseases/blood clots (especially so in women who are taking the pill and smoking).
- The exogenous (outside the body) supply of oestrogen increases the production of prostaglandins, which increase inflammation in the body. Subsequently, B vitamins are depleted in order to put out the fire. Unfortunately, if B vitamins are always being used to calm inflammation, other functions that require B vitamins are going to suffer, such as the ability to absorb nutrients in the digestive tract.
- Depletion of the following micronutrients and amino acids:
  - **Magnesium** – required for over 300 enzymatic processes in the body, so probably something you want an abundance of.
  - **Folate** – important for the synthesis and replication of DNA for tissue growth and essential before pregnancy and during the first twelve weeks to prevent neural tube

defects. Folate is also required to lower levels of homocysteine, thereby decreasing your risk of cardiovascular disease.

- **Vitamin B2 (riboflavin)** – essential for the production of ATP (or energy).
- **Vitamin B3 (niacin)** – helps the body to utilise carbs, proteins and fats, as well as help make cholesterol and steroid hormones.
- **Vitamin B6 (pyridoxine)** – important for the metabolism of amino acids and glycogen, production of haemoglobin and regulation of important neurotransmitters.
- **Vitamin B12 (cobalamin)** – essential for maintaining the integrity of the nervous system and for working with folate in methylation and reducing homocysteine.
- **Vitamin C** – acts as a major antioxidant in the body, and is key for the production of collagen fibres and other connective tissue components. It is also required for the production of corticosteroids, such as cortisol, and regulates iron absorption, storage and transport.
- **Tryptophan** – used to convert to serotonin, our happy hormone, and melatonin, our sleep hormone.
- **Tyrosine** – essential for the production of thyroid hormone, and therefore regulating metabolism.
- **Zinc** – important for growth, development, reproduction, immune function, insulin regulation and acts as an antioxidant.

❧ The pill can also throw off the balance of good versus bad bacteria in your digestive system, which can, in itself, cause issues with hormonal imbalance, absorption of nutrients, and digestion in general.

(Note: This is not an exhaustive list of the side effects of the pill, or the role of these nutrients that are depleted.)

# GETTING OFF THE PILL

If you decide you would like to stop taking the the pill, have a chat with your doctor and then use the following strategies to help support your body to come back into balance.

- Know that there is no perfect time to get off the pill. You do not have to wait until you go on the sugar pills. It is an artificial bleed anyway. Now is as good a time as any!
- Know that you might feel, act (and maybe look) a little worse before things get better. They WILL get better if you support your body to get back to balance. On the other hand, you might feel freakin' fantastic as soon as you stop taking it! Me? I had horrible headaches and upper back pain for about two weeks after – signs that my liver was suffering from a bit of a post-pill hangover.
- If you're sexually active and aren't already doing so, prepare yourself with alternative contraception (e.g. condoms).
- Consider supplementation to replenish your nutrient stores. Choose a good quality multi-vitamin, multi-mineral and probiotic. This is not necessary for forever; just to get things back online. If you're trying to conceive, I recommend waiting awhile after stopping the pill, and grab yourself a high quality prenatal supplement that has adequate folate (around 800 mcg) and iodine (150 mcg).
- Support your liver and detoxification. Hormones are metabolised and packaged up for elimination by the liver, so this baby needs to be in tip-top shape in order to get rid of all of the synthetic hormones in your body to start with a clean slate. I talk more about how to do this in Chapter 4: Happy gut = happy hormones.
- Manage your stress levels. The pill disrupts the pathway between the hypothalamus, the pituitary and the ovaries (known as the HPG axis, with G standing for gonadal, in case you cared). Stress also disrupts this pathway. Support the reconnection by incorporating stress management practices into each and every day. Chapter 7: Manage stress gives you more of the hows and whys on this one.
- Eat really good quality foods. Find more details in Chapter 5: Eat well.
- Be patient. It can take some time for things to get back on track. If you've been taking

the pill for ten years, don't expect things to be all fine and dandy within a month. Your body needs to rebuild and relearn. Be kind to yourself. It'll happen.

❧ Get in touch with your body's fertile signs and symptoms, such as cervical mucus and temperature changes.

I get that the pill is a personal choice that we are lucky to have as an option. But please, be aware that it is not a cure-all. If you have any hormonal imbalances, such as acne, endometriosis or PCOS, the pill will not fix these issues. It's not as simple as popping a pill. You need to address the underlying cause for long-term resolution.

## How do antibiotics mess up my hormones?

Antibiotics, while a godsend in many cases, can unfortunately have a devastating effect on your gut bacteria. This, in turn, has a negative impact on your overall digestion and, as you will learn about in Chapter 4: Happy gut = happy hormones, a healthy gut and optimal digestion are essential for proper hormone metabolism.

## What's my liver got to do with it?

Thanks for asking! Your liver plays a huge role in the detoxification of hormone metabolites (aka waste products). It helps to package these up into forms that are easy for your body to get rid of, via the gut. If your liver is suffering, detoxification is going to be poor, and you'll end up with toxic by-products (such as a harmful form of oestrogen) hanging around in your system and causing a ruckus. Flick to Chapter 4: Happy gut = happy hormones to learn more about the role of your liver and how to support it for happy hormones.

# I'm pregnant. Are my hormones messed up forever?

No, not forever, but they will be temporarily. In pregnancy, your progesterone and oestrogen go sky-high to help support a growing bubba. You have these abundant hormones to thank for your pregnancy glow. However, once the little one has made an entrance into the world (about three to five days after, actually), these hormones plummet *way* down, which is why the post-baby blues are common shortly after giving birth. It's also quite common for your thyroid to take a bit of a hit in pregnancy and post-partum. There's even a term for it – post-partum thyroiditis.

How can you mitigate these negative effects? Follow the strategies in this book, beautiful. And get some sleep (she says after a night of multiple wakings with her baby girl!) Just do what you can, and focus on the things you can control.

# What are these environmental toxins you speak of?

They are exactly as the name suggests – toxic products that are found in the environment around you. In the products you use, the water you drink, the house you live in, the air you breathe. Some are avoidable, some aren't. Many of these (such as BPA, phthalates, parabens and the like) are what we call endocrine disruptors because, you guessed it, they disrupt your endocrine (hormone) function. Choose natural products as much as possible, surround yourself with lots of greenery and drink lots of clean, filtered water.

# TESTING FOR OUT-OF-WHACK HORMONES

I don't recommend getting too caught up in test results, but there are some that you may want to consider looking into. Team up with a health practitioner who can go through your results with you.

## Blood tests

If you're up for getting a jab, some functions you may want to have tested include:

- Thyroid function – ask for TSH, T4 and T3 at the very least. If you have a healthcare professional who is open and willing, ask them if they would be happy to throw in 'reverse T3' and thyroid antibodies (they can indicate whether or not you have an autoimmune thyroid condition, such as Hashimoto's thyroiditis, or Grave's disease).
- Blood glucose control – insulin, HbA1C and fasting glucose.
- Sex hormone status – oestrogen, progesterone, testosterone, sex hormone binding globulin (SHBG) and dehydroepiandrosterone. (Say what now? Just ask for DHEA – it's a precursor to oestrogen and progesterone.)
- Liver function tests.
- Nutritional status – folate, vitamin B12, full iron panel, vitamin D, iodine (best to test this through a urine sample), homocysteine (if this is elevated, or if you are having trouble conceiving, request to see if you are a carrier of the methylenetetrahydrofolate reductase (or MTHFR, gene mutation).
- C-Reactive protein (a measure of inflammation in the body).

## Saliva tests

If you're interested in knowing what is happening with your cortisol levels, it is best to check this with multiple saliva tests throughout the day. This is because your cortisol levels change throughout the day (ideally high in the morning to help wake you up, and low in the evening to encourage a restful sleep).

These tests can be a bit pricey. But if you're cashed up and into checking out what is going on in your body then go for it.

# Stool tests

Yep. Poop tests. While this might sound really unappealing to you, stool tests can be incredibly valuable, especially if you are suffering from digestive issues. You won't be testing hormone levels with stool tests, but if your gut function is sub-optimal, chances are your hormones will not be that stellar either.

If you're keen, ask your health practitioner for a CSA (comprehensive stool analysis). This includes parasitology, which can show whether or not you have some not-so-friendly bugs living in your tummy.

The downside of stool tests? You have to poop in a cup, and the test can be quite costly.

## Recap time

- ❧ Hormone imbalance can present in many ways, from skin issues, to emotional outbursts, infertility, constipation, anxiety, heavy periods, no periods, facial hair and more!
- ❧ Several key factors that contribute to hormonal imbalance include stress, exercise, the pill, antibiotics, poor gut health, dodgy liver function, pregnancy and environmental toxins. It's your lucky day, as we cover off how to avoid these bad-boys in the coming chapters.
- ❧ There is no ideal time to get off the pill – now is as good as any!
- ❧ If you're up for it, you can test the hormones in your blood, saliva and your poop.

So now you know how hormones can either boost you up or bring you down, let's move on to how to ensure everything is *en pointe* to help you feel like one very saucy lady.

# HAPPY GUT = HAPPY HORMONES

*All disease begins in the gut.*
– Hippocrates

Ahh, Hippocrates. How right he was so many, many years ago. How on earth did we get so off track? When did we start assuming that nothing is fixable without drugs? Don't get me wrong, modern medicine is awesome, and I am grateful for it, but many issues, especially hormonal issues, could and should be first addressed by looking at the root cause of the issue, and often this can all come back to your gut.

What does your gut have to do with your hormones? Everything! Happy gut = happy hormones! But in case you want a little more …

To start with, your gut is where you break down your food and absorb all of your nutrients. These nutrients are essential for providing the building blocks for, and ensuring proper function of, all of your hormones. You'll learn more about this in the next chapter. If you have a healthy gut, you'll get the most out of your food, and your hormones will thank you for it. If you have an unhealthy gut, your hormones will not reap the benefits of this good nutrition and will become imbalanced, leading to all of the not-so-pleasant symptoms that come along with cranky hormones, which you read about in Chapter 3: Hormones going haywire.

At the other end (literally), your gut needs to be in optimal working condition in order to eliminate excess hormones that have been used by the body and no longer wanted. When everything is working well, they will be excreted without an issue. When you have gut issues such as constipation, you'll be more likely to reabsorb these (now harmful) hormones back into your system, leading to imbalances (and even an increased risk of cancer).

In this chapter, you'll learn all about the things to avoid that contribute to an unhealthy gut, as well as what this might look like, literally. We are going to talk poop 'cos it's important. And, of course, we'll delve into simple ways to flip the switch back to a well-nourished, healthy gut, which will ensure your hormones are happy and balanced.

# WHERE IS THIS GUT?

I suspect there are quite a few differing ideas of the gut. Let's clear things up with a basic outline of what the gut does. Your entire gut is, essentially, a hollow tube that runs from your mouth to your anus – top to tail, so to speak. What you put in your mouth and isn't absorbed in the intestines will simply pass straight out the other end.

Did you know that digestion actually starts in the mouth? This is something to keep in mind, as many of us do not chew our food, which can lead to digestive issues downstream. Chewing helps break down food mechanically, but also triggers the release of saliva, which contains enzymes to help break down our food chemically. Also, when we chew our food, this sends messages to our brain that food is incoming, so it can prepare the appropriate hormones (such as insulin) to help our body utilise the goodness and also tell you when you have had enough to eat.

We're not ducks, ladies. There's a reason we have teeth – use them. Chew. Your. Food. It could be the single thing that helps with things like bloating, constipation, gas, reflux and even overeating.

Then we move onto the stomach. Once in here, the food we've eaten (and chewed sufficiently, right?) is attacked by hydrochloric acid – super-strong acid that is released by the cells of the stomach. It is incredibly important to have sufficient stomach acid as this turns our food into mush (called chyme) and also creates a pH gradient, so when said mush passes out of the stomach, the acidity triggers the release of digestive enzymes that further disintegrate the food into tiny molecules that can be absorbed in the intestines.

Low stomach acid is a *huge* issue for many peeps that I see. What causes it? A few things. Think about whether any of these apply to you.

- Chronic stress.
- Acid-lowering drugs, such as Gaviscon and Mylanta – the kind you would be prescribed for reflux.
- H. pylori infection.
- Age – not really avoidable, unfortunately.
- Vegetarian/vegan diet.

So it makes sense to eliminate these factors to help boost stomach acid production. Plus, you can throw in a few of the following to help you out.

- Apple cider vinegar – 1 teaspoon in some water 30 minutes before meals.
- Dandelion root tea – 30 minutes before meals.
- Bitter herbs – such as fennel, ginger, wormwood and milk thistle.
- Fermented foods – build up to 1 tablespoon with each meal (see Chapter 5: Eat well)
- A little pineapple pre-meal – this tropical goodie contains bromelain, an enzyme that helps with protein digestion.
- Supplemental digestive enzymes, ox bile and hydrochloric acid – best to work with a practitioner on this one to make sure you actually need them.

Next are the intestines ... small and large. Our intestines are vital to our overall health as this is where the absorption (or lack thereof) of nutrients occurs (mostly in the small intestine, large intestines absorb water and pack everything up to be pooped out). When your gut is nice and healthy with the intestinal lining intact, teeny tiny parts of nutrients (think amino acids from proteins, sugars from carbohydrates and fatty acids from fats) can cross over into our blood stream (through something called tight junctions) to be utilised throughout the body (including the making and functioning of hormones). Meanwhile, larger and foreign bits and pieces will hang out in the intestines and then be passed out as waste. Good stuff.

# THE BUGS IN YOUR BELLY

Now, what's more important than the gut itself are the critters that actually live inside our gut. You might have heard these referred to as bacteria, probiotics, or even (for the nerdy science-minded show-offs) the microbiome.

A microbiome is the ecological community of commensal, symbiotic and pathogenic microorganisms that literally share our body space.

I think we should use the term 'share' lightly, because they actually comprise 90 per cent of the cells on and in our body, whereas only 10 per cent are human cells. Not exactly sharing the space now, is it?

Let's just clarify one thing, though. These bacteria inhabit our skin, vaginal canal, mouth and respiratory tract; however, the largest proportion hang out in the large intestine (the colon/gut). Because this is where most of these little babies are, the gut microbiome is what we will focus on – the place where you will get the most bang for your buck, so to speak.

There are 500–1000 species of bacteria in the gut (and more being discovered all the time); however, they mostly belong to two families – Firmicutes and Bacteroidetes. Remember that, I'll test you later. Not really, but it is relevant info.

So where do these little critters come from?

# THERE'S A HOLE IN MY GUT, DEAR LIZA, DEAR LIZA

When the integrity of our intestines is compromised, the tight junctions, which act as gate-keepers to our body, can become not-so-tight (with the help of a little protein called zonulin), and let these larger and unwanted bits and bobs pass through into our bloodstream. This is often referred to as a leaky gut and is problematic as when these foreign particles sneak through the barriers and get into our bloodstream, they trigger the immune system to say 'Hey! You're not supposed to be in here! Get out!' Subsequently, your immune system attempts to get rid of them so they don't do any damage. They are kind of like drunk, unwanted party crashers.

What can then happen is your immune system can get a little confused, or trigger-happy, and some of your body's own cells can get caught in the fire – friendly fire, if you will. This then can lead to widespread inflammation and possibly even autoimmune conditions such as rheumatoid arthritis, psoriasis and Hashimoto's thyroiditis. Not to mention this inflammation is going to be throwing your hormones into absolute chaos. So it's kinda important to maintain the integrity of your gut lining through eating a healthy diet (including super-foods to nourish the gut – see page 82), avoiding dodgy food-like substances (gluten has been implicated with triggering the release of zonulin and causing the tight junctions to open wider than they should), and managing your stress and sleep.

# From mum to bub

We used to think that bub's gut was essentially sterile until birth, but new research is suggesting that mum's gut bacteria can actually influence her child's gut flora in utero. This highlights the importance of mum's diet during pregnancy in having a positive influence on her child's health.

Within twenty minutes of birth, a baby's microbial implant is established and will reflect the method of birth. If he is born vaginally, then the gut flora will reflect mum's vaginal flora. If he is born via C-section, the flora will be more like mum's skin and the hospital environment

Fun fact: breast milk contains oligosaccharides (sugars) that are unable to be digested by the baby; however, they provide food for the beneficial bacteria to proliferate, which will help in the development of a strong, resilient system. How cool is that? Nature's wisdom, eh?

# The environment

Think soil, animals, other humans. Remember the days, before we all became hyper-hygienic, when babies were allowed to eat dirt and worms and it wasn't such a big issue if a dog licked their face? Maybe that all happened for a reason ... again, helping to build a robust immune system.

# Food

If you're eating a whole-foods diet then you can acquire bacteria from your food – probiotic rich foods to inoculate the gut; prebiotic rich foods to feed the good bugs. A little dirt on your veggies to provide soil-based organisms. We'll chat about probiotics and prebiotics a little later, don't stress.

# WHAT DO GUT BACTERIA DO?

A better question might be 'what don't they do?' For the sake of brevity (and so you don't fall asleep), I'm not going to go deep into the science, but research has shown that the gut microbiome plays a role in the following (to name a few).

## Digestive health

- ❧ Normal, healthy gastro-intestinal function, which as I have mentioned, is essential for healthy hormone function.
- ❧ The renewal of intestinal epithelial cells (the lining of the intestines – and a hugely important barrier system between the outside world and your blood stream). You want this barrier to be intact. If it becomes leaky, this can lead to a persistent state of inflammation, which will leave you feeling pretty cruddy and increase your risk of hormone imbalance and chronic disease).
- ❧ Fat metabolism (bacteria can modify bile acids, which are essential for fat digestion, and fats are super-important for building hormones).

People with irritable bowel syndrome (IBS) and irritable bowel disease (IBD), including Chrohn's disease and ulcerative colitis), have shown markedly different microbiomes than healthy populations, hinting at the role of these little creatures in modulating the health of your gut.

# Mental health

You know when you get butterflies in your tummy, or a gut feeling, or the nervous runs? That is a clear indication that there is a connection between the gut and the brain. And this has been established in the research – it's called the gut–brain axis and something called the vagus nerve connects the two systems into a two-way communication mecca.

Here's a nice little diagram of all of the bits and bobs in your body that the vagus nerve has its mitts on. Missing from the image is your noggin, which is obviously a vital part of the picture.

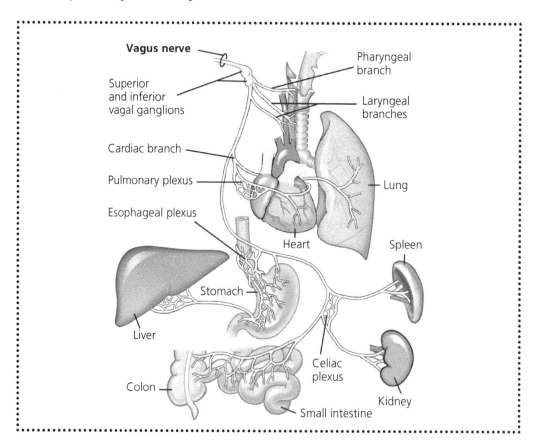

Our bacteria also play a role in our tendency towards depression and anxiety. How so? Ninety-five per cent of serotonin (your happy brain chemical) is produced in your gut, and your bacteria modulate the stuff.

## Skin health

It has been proposed that there is a gut–brain–skin axis. Woah! Skin inflammation (skinflammation?) has been associated with an imbalance of gut bacteria and intestinal permeability, which manifests as acne, eczema, rosacea, psoriasis and all the not-so-fun stuff. Not to mention if your gut health causes your hormones to go all whacky, you'll be more likely to have skin issues, such as acne with PCOS when testosterone levels soar.

## Immunity

Seventy to eighty per cent of the body's immune cells are in the gut. Gut bacteria and the immune cells talk to each other to produce either pro- or anti-inflammatory chemicals. Freaky!

## Weight

You know how I said that Firmicutes and Bacteroidetes were important? (You'd blanked that, hadn't you?) Studies have found that more of the former in relation to the latter can contribute to weight gain - possibly through extracting more kilojoules from your food. So if you have more Firmicutes than I do, and we eat the same apple, you will probably absorb more kilojoules from said apple. Cheeky buggers!

## Synthesis of vitamins

Most vitamins are required to be supplied through what you put in your gob – through whole foods, such as fresh veggies, fruit, eggs and the like.

However, there are a few exceptions that can actually be made by our bacteria – clever little sods, they are! Most notably, these little critters are able to magically whip up B vitamins and vitamin K.

# WHAT THE BUGS IN YOUR BELLY DON'T LIKE

There are quite a few things that upset your gut bacteria that, ideally, you should avoid (sorry to be a party-pooper), or at least minimise to keep your gut running like a well-oiled machine.

1  Smoking – just another reason to ditch the cancer sticks.
2  Stress can throw out the balance by increasing pathogenic (bad) bacteria and decreasing beneficial bacteria – more reason to take a chill pill! See Chapter 7: Manage stress.
3  Excessive alcohol intake can contribute to bacterial overgrowth in the small intestine (out of bounds for the bugs; their hood is lower down in the large intestine) – this can lead to a leaky gut whereby bacteria and other uninvited guests can get into our bloodstream and cause widespread damage in our body.
4  Antibiotics – anti = against; biota = living organisms. Self-explanatory, I think. But if you do need to take antibiotics (and sometimes they ARE necessary), or if you have done so in the past, be sure to pay extra attention to nourishing your gut bugs to help get things back on track.

**5** Oral contraceptive pill – your daily dose of contraceptive hormones could be increasing your levels of pathogenic (bad) bacteria, leading to an imbalance in gut bugs and increased problems with hormones.

**6** Proton pump inhibitors (prescribed for reflux) – PPIs work by increasing the pH of your stomach acid (thereby making it less acidic), which has a downstream effect of encouraging the growth of bad bacteria, as well as decreasing overall microbial diversity.

**7** Excessive hygiene – let your kids eat worms and throw away the antibacterial wipes/soaps/ liquids.

**8** Poor diet–
  • Processed foods are devoid of bacteria.
  • Omega 6 fatty acids (as in those found in dodgy, heart-healthy vegetable oils) have been shown to disrupt intestinal flora and increase inflammation.
  • Artificial sweeteners have been shown to worsen glucose intolerance (our ability, or lack thereof, to deal with carbohydrates). Aspartame, often found in diet soft drinks, can modify populations of bacteria and can get converted to methanol and formaldehyde! Very bad. Avoid!

**9** Jet lag – not really avoidable in our jet-setting world. Pay extra attention to nourishing your gut bacteria if you're a frequent-flyer.

**10** Obviously life-saving in many cases, but caesarean births have been shown to increase risk of allergies, asthma and obesity.

# WHAT THE BUGS DO LIKE

While there is quite an extensive list of things that our gut bacteria don't like (fussy little buggers), there are quite a few things that can really help to nourish them. Try to engage in as many of the following as possible and expect to be shown a little love in return, in the form of a healthy, well-functioning digestive system and perfect hormone balance.

## Organic whole-foods

These are foods that are produced in healthy soil and free of antibiotics, chemicals and hormones. Studies on conventional farms (that use antibiotics as growth promoters in livestock) have shown that the chickens (and humans eating them) carry antibiotic-resistant bacteria. Those on organic farms do not. Antibiotic resistance has been named as one of the most significant global threats to public health. As much as we should not overuse antibiotics as they mess up our gut, they can be truly life-saving. If they stop working, we may actually be in the situation where we could die from a simple infection. Not cool.

## Fermented foods

Yum! Sauerkraut, beet kvass, kombucha, kefir, yoghurt, kimchi, pickles, the list goes on. Take your pick or mix 'n' match to inoculate your body with beneficial bacteria that will help to nourish your gut and, in turn, your entire body. Check out Chapter 9: Recipes to see how to make these goodies.

## Probiotic supplements

I prefer to encourage intake of probiotics from whole-food sources, however, there is a tonne of research showing how different probiotic strains can improve a myriad of ills such as strengthening the intestinal barrier and immunity, reducing stress hormones, improving anxiety and depression, improve and prevent eczema, decreasing gestational diabetes, and improving adverse digestive symptoms. Need I say more?

## Prebiotics

These are the darlings of the health world right now. These are the non-digestible, but fermentable, foods that have beneficial effects by stimulating the growth and activity of bacteria in the colon. Ergo, they feed your good bugs. Find them in unripe bananas, green banana flour (yes, it's a thing, and makes pretty tasty muffins – see page 243 for the Banana Flour Carrot Muffins), cold potato/white rice (cook it first, please!), acacia fibre, potato starch, asparagus, garlic, artichokes, onions, carrots, tomatoes, leeks and radish.

## Vaginal birth and breastfeeding

C-section rates are at one in three, with elective C-sections on the increase. It is preferable, however for the health of your child or yourself, not to have a C-section. Obviously if that isn't possible or if you were born via C-section and/or not breastfed, just focus on what you *can* do instead.

## Faecal microbiota transplant

Yep, transplanting healthy poop into an unhealthy colon. This is relatively new stuff, but is showing promising results, having been so far effective 82–100 of the time in the treatment of the pathogenic bacteria, *C. difficile*. There is speculation that it could be helpful for many other conditions, such as IBS, IBD, autoimmunity, neurological disorders, obesity, chronic fatigue and autism. Watch this space! Oh, and please do not try this at home!

So there you have it, a little snapshot of how incredible the bugs in your belly are and what a wide-reaching impact they can have on your health. What you have read here only just scratches the surface of this fascinating topic! Now go forth and allow your bacteria to flourish so you do too.

# THE END OF THE LINE: LET'S TALK BOWELS

And by bowels, I mean your large intestine (aka colon). As you read previously, most nutrients (vitamins, minerals, sugars, amino acids and fatty acids) are absorbed in the small intestine. As food moves through the large intestine, water is absorbed from the digested food matter to form waste products/your stool (fancy term for poop). Peristalsis (nerd-speak for muscle contractions) pushes the poop toward the rectum at which stage it is solid, because most of the water has been absorbed.

So, have you checked out your poop lately? This will probably sound like an odd question, and I can already feel some of you screwing your noses up as you read this, but stay with me, this is important!

What comes out of your body as faecal waste can be a very good indicator of how well things are functioning inside your body, and specifically, in your gut. That's right, you can go to a doctor and get a whole bunch of fancy blood tests, or ask them their professional opinion, or you could just start to check out what goes into the toilet bowl after passing a number two.

# Types of poop

Healthy poop is a sign of a healthy gut. And a healthy gut is a must for happy hormones. So while you might be thinking, 'Why do I need to check out my poop?', keep in mind that your poop provides a good window into how well your hormones are going to work.

So what are you looking for? Here are some things you might see going on with your floaters. Time to become a poop detective! Sounds fun, right? Have you ever heard of the Bristol Stool Chart? No? It's a chart that we health professionals use to classify your poop! Lucky us! What you're looking for, ideally, is a type 4 – smooth as a sausage. Type 3 and 5 are okay, too. Anything lower than 3 is constipation. Anything higher than 5 is diarrhoea. There you go. Poop 101.

| Bristol stool chart | | |
|---|---|---|
| Type 1 | | Separate hard lumps, like nuts (hard to pass) |
| Type 2 | | Sausage-shaped but lumpy |
| Type 3 | | Like a sausage but with cracks on its surface |
| Type 4 | | Like a sausage or snake, smooth and soft |
| Type 5 | | Soft blobs with clear-cut edges (passed easily) |
| Type 6 | | Fluffy pieces with ragged edges, a mushy stool |
| Type 7 | | Watery, no solid pieces, Entirely liquid |

A few other things that you might see in the loo, post-poop include the following.

**Oily slick, frothy, floating:** If you're noticing this, then chances are you are not digesting fats properly. This is quite common when you go from a low fat diet to eating more healthy fats, as your gallbladder, which helps to digest fats by releasing bile, needs a little time to catch on to the changes. You might need to work on chewing your food more mindfully and slowly. You also might benefit from some digestive support, such as supplemental digestive enzymes, or consuming bitter products prior to meal times.

**Green:** Probably just a result of eating lots of greens, and nothing to worry about. As you were.

**Red:** First of all, don't freak out. Stop and think, 'Have I eaten fresh beetroot in the last 24–48 hours?' If the answer is 'yes', then there's your answer. If the answer is 'no', and it looks more like blood in the stool, then you should head to your doc at your earliest convenience. This usually indicates a problem with your colon, rectum and anus and should be checked out ASAP, just to be safe. Comprenez-vous?

**Black, tarry and/or sticky:** Again, stop and think first – have you been eating lots of licorice or blueberries? Perhaps taking an iron supplement? These can cause your poop to go quite dark. If it's a no to those goodies, then head to your doctor for a check-up as there may be some bleeding going on in your digestive system, which needs prompt attention. Go! Now!

**Brown:** Congratulations. Your poop is of normal hue. (You probably didn't need a book to tell you that, though, did you?)

**Hard to pass:** Hello, constipation! Constipation can be a result of your large intestine absorbing too much water, or if the muscle contractions are slow/ sluggish, it can cause the stool to move through too slowly, resulting in dry, hard-to-pass stools. See 'Getting poop out: ten great ways to find relief' on page 79 if this is a problem for you.

Not only is constipation uncomfortable and distressing, it can cause health problems. Products that should be eliminated on a regular basis (such as hormones and by-products of medications), may be reabsorbed by the colon, leading to hormonal imbalance and general toxicity.

There could be a number of other things causing you to be blocked up such as:

❧ Inadequate vegetable intake – we need fibre to bulk up the stool and improve movement of said stool through the digestive system out into the loo.

❧ Low-carb diets – cutting out carbs might have a negative impact on digestive function by starving the bugs in your belly, which actually make up quite a large proportion of your poop.

❧ Inadequate water intake – when your body is well hydrated, less water will need to be absorbed from your large intestine and therefore this extra moisture will make passing a stool a lot easier

❧ Lack of exercise – movement, especially walking and twisting, can encourage peristalsis – a fancy term for movement of the bowel to encourage the poop through the passage.

❧ Stress and/or anxiety – when you are stressed, your rest and digest system is shut off. Pooping is part of digestion so unfortunately, when you're locked and loaded in that fight or flight mode, your stool is going to stall! How's that for a sentence full of alliteration?

❧ Food intolerances – I'm looking at you, dairy and gluten! Some of you might also experience intolerances to something called FODMAPs – these are certain types of sugars found in a range of foods. It's possible you could benefit from following a low-FODMAP diet to improve the flow of things. I would suggest you work with a health practitioner on this one though, as the diet can be a little restrictive.

**Incomplete evacuation:** Do you get off the loo feeling a little like, 'Was that it? I think I need to do more!', but can't pass any more? This could be related to constipation, or it could be something more sinister, such as irritable bowel syndrome or coeliac disease. Go get a check-up, beauty, just to be safe.

**Undigested food:** This one might also be loose and watery. Check one – are you chewing your food well, in a relaxed environment? No? Okay – start there. Yes? This could be another case of inadequate digestive fire, which might require supplementation. Alternatively there could be something going on with your colon, resulting in poor digestion and food in the poop.

**Alternating bouts of diarrhoea and constipation:** How annoying is this one! I have been here, so I get it. This is tied in with irritable bowel syndrome and food intolerances, most specifically to gluten and dairy – why not try 30 days without them and see if you notice an improvement? The other possibility is a parasitic infection (fun!), which you will need to get a stool test to determine. Work with a health professional on this one: I can't imagine you want to (or know how to) collect and analyse your own poop in your at-home lab aka kitchen – eww!

**Smells really bad:** Let's be honest. No-one's poop smells like roses. However, if you are almost passing out from the fumes every time you do a number two then something else could be going on. It's most likely a lack of beneficial bacteria, but it also could be excess consumption of spicy foods and/or protein. (Note, it is rare that I find a female who eats too much protein, so this one is unlikely.)

**Diarrhoea:** There are many causes of diarrhoea:

- ❧ Infections – viral, bacterial or parasitic.
- ❧ Food poisoning.
- ❧ Malabsorption (poor absorption in the small intestines) – usually related to lactose intolerance, coeliac disease or gluten intolerance, cow's milk protein intolerance, or a reaction to other foods that don't mesh well with your constitution.
- ❧ Inflammatory bowel disease – such as Crohn's and ulcerative colitis.
- ❧ Medications such as antibiotics, laxatives or chemotherapy.

# GETTING POOP OUT – TEN GREAT WAYS TO GET RELIEF

So what can you do about the poop that won't appear? Try these out when you get a little stuck (pun intended!):

1 Drink more water – I know this sounds very obvious and not sexy at all, but if you are dehydrated, chances are your poop will be too. The general guidelines are about 33 ml/kg of body weight. So, for example, if you weigh 60 kilograms, your water intake should be around 2 litres a day, maybe more if you're sweating your little butt off. Maybe try mixing up plain water with chamomile tea, which can help relax the smooth muscles of your large intestine. And try to keep liquids away from meals, as this can dilute digestive enzymes needed to break down your food.

2 Exercise – go for a walk early in the morning, preferably up a hill. Physical activity encourages peristalsis of the bowels and gets things moving.

3 Deep belly breathing – start your day (still lying in bed) by taking ten breaths deep into your belly. With your hands on your tummy, feel your abdomen rise and fall with your breath. This will help to activate your parasympathetic nervous system (aka your rest and digest system). See Chapter 8: Be Kind for more stress-busting, poop-encouraging tips.

4 Consume fermented foods – foods such as sauerkraut, beet kvass, kefir, full-fat yoghurt and kombucha are fantastic sources of probiotics and can improve gut function, especially constipation, by repopulating your gut with beneficial bacteria. Start with small amounts and build up. If you're not keen on fermented foods, consider a high quality probiotic supplement.

5 Make sure you eat enough carbohydrates – this one is three-fold. 1) Your thyroid gland requires carbohydrates/insulin to convert the inactive to the active form of thyroid hormone. Without sufficient thyroid hormone, metabolism slows. Constipation is a common symptom of a sluggish thyroid. Get it checked out, if you are concerned. 2) Carbohydrates are food for your gut bacteria (prebiotic) – insufficient carbs and you are essentially starving these little babies in your belly that make up quite a large

proportion of your stool weight. 3) Carbs (the fruit and veg variety) provide fibre to bulk up the stool and also get it moving along.

6  Squat – and I don't mean with weights (although you should do that anyway). The ideal position to be in when you are evacuating your bowels (that sounded professional, didn't it?) is the squat position. If you're all blocked up, you could consider getting a squatty potty (or just pile up some old-school phone books so your knees are slightly higher than your hips when you're on the dunny). We aren't really designed to sit on toilets to poop – it's just another one of those conveniences that have turned out to be not so convenient.

7  Consume adequate fats – so many of my clients see resolution in their constipation symptoms once they ditch their low-fat diet and start including nourishing fats such as coconut oil, olive oil, avocado and butter. Speaking of butter, it can help with the production of butyric acid, which is beneficial for gut health. Winning!

8  Have 1 teaspoon of apple cider vinegar 30 minutes before meals – it helps stimulate digestion. Bitters such as dandelion, mustard greens and endive can do the same. I like to have a dandelion tea an hour or so before meals to help get the juices (digestive) flowing.

9  Chew. Your. Food. Seriously – don't eat on the run. Sit down and really chew your food. Digestion starts in the mouth, so don't skip this vital step.

10 Vitamin C and magnesium supplements can be helpful for poop problems. I find magnesium especially helpful as it works by relaxing the smooth muscle (and encourages sleep).

# How often do you go?

What I'm talking about here is your bowel transit time, or how long your stool takes to get from station A (your mouth) to station B (your lavatory). In a perfect world, it should take about 12–24 hours, so ideally, you should be going on a daily basis, if not more than once a day. Any longer than two days and you're looking at constipation and potential health issues and hormone imbalances.

How can you check this transit time? Pretty easily, actually. Here's what you do:

- ❧ Consume either 1 cup of corn, 1 cup of beetroot or a few tablespoons of sesame seeds. Make a note of what time you have eaten said food (this is station A).
- ❧ Note down the time when said food shows up in your loo (station B).
- ❧ Count the number of hours between station A and station B and voila! There's your transit time!

If your transit time is much longer than 24 hours, try the suggestions for constipation earlier in this chapter to help work things out. (Loving all the puns in here, yet?). Anything faster than ten hours is also problematic, as this means you are probably not absorbing all of the goodness from your food and there could be some issues with your digestive system. Go see your friendly health practitioner and see what the jig is.

## Some final remarks on the poop front

Other than checking out what your poop actually looks like and making sure it is looking healthy, also be mindful if you are experiencing any of the following, which could also indicate that your digestive system needs some TLC:

- ❧ gas – at either end. Yes, I mean burps and bottom burps. (This is what my niece calls them. Sounds nicer than farts, don't you think?)
- ❧ bloating
- ❧ indigestion
- ❧ reflux
- ❧ abdominal pain
- ❧ gurgling
- ❧ smelly breath.

# SUPER-FOODS TO NOURISH THE GUT

Often when we think of super-foods, we put them in the icing-on-the-cake basket. Instead, I would encourage you to put the following goodies in your daily must-have basket. (Don't worry – they're cheap!) Enjoying these on a regular basis will ensure your gut (and hormones) stay in their happy place. If you have a gut issue already, then you will need to be even more diligent about incorporating these foods into your daily intake.

## Fermented foods

Are you thinking, 'What on earth are fermented foods? Are they mouldy? Gross!' Well, yes and no. Fermentation involves leaving certain types of foods in a warm environment where said foods are then transformed through enzymatic reactions, creating an abundance of friendly bacteria (probiotics).

Fermented foods have long been a part of traditional cultures. Not only is fermentation great for your health, it's also a way to preserve foods. Very handy when you don't have a refrigerator in your cave to stop them from going off.

Not only are fermented foods wonderful for boosting your good bacteria population, but when you ferment foods, you also increase the vitamin and mineral content. Quite significantly in some cases. Take sauerkraut (fermented cabbage), for example. The fermented form has 100–300 per cent more vitamin C than the raw form. Win!

A few fermented foods you might want to consider getting into your daily diet include:

❧ Sauerkraut – fermented cabbage.
❧ Kimchi – spicy fermented veggies.
❧ Kefir – this is traditionally fermented milk, but can also be made with water or coconut water (VERY yummy).

- Yoghurt and cheese – fermented milk.
- Wine – fermented grapes (sold on this one?).
- Kombucha – fermented tea.

Start small and increase gradually. Also, the more variety you can get with your fermented goodies, the better. (I suspect many of you have already experimented with wine and cheese.) I find that kombucha is a nice one to start with (see my recipe on page 231).

# Resistant starch

Resistant starch (RS) is the portion of starch that resists digestion as it passes through the small intestine to the large intestine, where it becomes a fermentable feast for your good bacteria.

Some other potential beneficial effects of RS (other than nourishing your good bacteria) include:

- Improved blood sugar management – which could be helpful for those with pre-diabetes, diabetes, metabolic syndrome or PCOS (polycystic ovarian syndrome).
- Better bowel health – something to consider if you suffer from constipation, irritable bowel disease (such as ulcerative colitis) or diverticulitis.
- More favourable blood lipid profile – I'm talking cholesterol and triglycerides here.
- Increased satiety – which can possibly aid in weight loss and weight management.
- Production of short chain fatty acids (SCFAs) – such as butyrate, propionate and acetate – these SCFAs provide fuel for the cells of the colon wall and increase colonic blood flow.
- Improved immune function.

So where can we find this good stuff? Lots of places:

- Green bananas (you can throw these into a smoothie), and green banana flour.

- Cooked and cooled white potatoes (they must be cooled, which causes something called retrogradation, which makes the starch in the potato resistant to digestion. Hot 'taters won't cut it, though they are nevertheless delicious and should still be enjoyed!
- Cooked and cooled white rice (as for potatoes).
- Legumes such as beans, lentils and chickpeas (if you can tolerate these, it might be worth incorporating them into your diet on the odd occasion to promote gut health).
- Fibre supplements such as inulin, acacia fibre and potato starch (best to work with someone in the know when using these as they can cause some not-so-pleasant side effects if not taken appropriately).
- Buckwheat flour – buckwheat is a fruit seed that can be tolerated by people who can't eat wheat flour.

# Carbs

Another reason not to avoid them. They provide food for your belly bugs. In fact, I see women with huge digestive issues (and consequently hormone issues) as a result of inappropriately following a low-carb diet for too long.

# Bone broth

Boil up some bones and have a mug, or use it as a base for soups and stews just like your grandma used to do. The glycine and gelatin in bone broth are wonderful gut-healers. See page 239 for the recipe.

# Breastmilk

Don't worry, I'm not suggesting that you hit up your local breastmilk bank (or accost a breastfeeding mum) and put this liquid gold in your smoothies. I put this here so those of you who are pregnant, or looking to get pregnant in the future, understand that breast milk provides an abundance of beneficial bugs to your baby, which can help establish healthy, lifelong digestive function.

# COLONICS

A colonic is where a tube is inserted into your nether regions (of the bottom variety), and warm water is flushed through your colon. It's hydrotherapy for your colon, which is why it is often referred to as colon hydrotherapy.

I'm not going to lie. I'm not a huge fan of colonics on a regular basis. The main reason is that in the process of clearing out the bad, they also wipe out the good, in this case, your good bacteria. (This is why they offer you a token probiotic post-colonic.) And when you wipe out your good bacteria, you essentially throw off your digestive balance, potentially leading to even more gut issues.

Also, many places that offer colonics claim to improve 'nutrient absorption'. Here, I call BS! Colonics work by flushing out your large intestine, with the fluid stopping at your cecum (which is the intersection between your large and small intestine).

Very few nutrients are absorbed in the large intestine. The majority of nutrient absorption occurs in the small intestine. So how, then, if the colonic activity stops before it reaches the small intestine, can it improve nutrient absorption?

A colonic might be useful if you haven't passed a bowel motion in a long time. It might do you some good to flush things out. As mentioned previously, if waste products sit in your large intestine for too long, substances that should be excreted may be reabsorbed into the body and cause issues, especially hormonal imbalances (such as oestrogen dominance).

So maybe get it out, then address why it was staying in there for so long, as opposed to relying on regular colonics to empty your bowels.

# YOUR LIVER AND DETOXIFICATION

Your liver is your number one organ of detoxification. But you already knew that, right? It's responsible for packing up waste products and getting them ready for elimination.

Your liver is also responsible for a lot of hormone metabolism and so, if you are not showing your liver a little love, you could potentially be contributing to hormone imbalance.

How so? Hormones, once used, become waste products. Yep, we use them and then we toss them. We need our liver to package up these hormone waste products and help the body to get rid of them. Without this process working efficiently, we can potentially fail to excrete these toxins, which will then get reabsorbed into the circulation, causing imbalances and wreaking havoc. This is a biggy with oestrogen dominance. Especially if you aren't pooping well, oestrogen will take that opportunity to sneak back into your body.

Your body is going through a process of detoxification all the time. Not just when you decide to do a juice cleanse/clean eating/30-day challenge/water fast. It's pretty complex, too. I'm going to try my best to break it down for you here, but just be aware that we are learning more and more about these bodily processes each and every day, and are discovering that a number of factors can affect your ability to properly detoxify, such as:

- Food
- Lifestyle
- Environment
- Medications
- Genetics (this is a tricky one, as some genetic defects can greatly affect detoxification).

# What is detoxification??

Basically, detoxification is the process of transforming toxins that enter (via medications, skin care products, air, food, etc) or accumulate in our body (as a by-product of metabolism, hormones, etc) into waste products that can be readily excreted (via poop or pee).

Most detoxification occurs in the liver; however, some occurs in the wall of the intestines (or gut), and a little also in our lungs, brain and kidneys, so it is important to look after all of our organ systems, as opposed to just focusing on our lovely livers.

If you are not detoxifying properly, you can experience an array of symptoms such as skin breakouts, poor digestion, hormonal imbalance, migraines, emotional outbursts and achy muscles and joints.

# The three phases of detoxification

Now this is the technical part, but I'm going to try to minimise my science mumbo-jumbo as best I can to make it easier to understand (hopefully).

## Phase I detoxification

Phase I begins the detoxification process with an enzyme family known as Cytochrome P450 (other enzymes are also involved, but this is the big daddy). P450 uses oxygen and NADH (the active form of the vitamin niacin) to add a reactive hydroxyl group to the toxin to be excreted. This makes it more water-soluble, easier to excrete, and less likely to be reabsorbed.

Phase I detoxification does not require much nutritional support and may actually increase during fasting, which forces toxins from fat and lean tissue into the circulation. This increased detoxification might sound just dandy to you, but please note – phase I detox often creates compounds that are more toxic than the original toxins. These compounds have the ability to increase oxidative stress and inflammation, potentially damaging DNA and proteins. Not good.

Because oxidation increases in this step, it's a good idea to always include an abundance of antioxidants from fresh, bright and colourful veggies and fruits. Eat the rainbow!

## Phase II detoxification

Phase II is all about reducing the activity and toxicity of the compound that was formed in phase I, and combining it with hydrophilic (water-loving) compounds. This allows for a speedy elimination.

There are a number of enzymes and processes that can take place during phase II, which basically refer to what the toxic compound is combined with:

- Glucuronidation
- Sulfation
- Glutathione conjugation (this baby is your body's number one antioxidant)
- Amino acid conjugation
- Acetylation
- Methylation.

If phase II detox is inhibited in any way (i.e. insufficient nutrition) or phase I is up-regulated without a simultaneous increase in phase II (i.e. fasting with insufficient nutrition), then you may find yourself up a creek without a paddle.

## Phase III detoxification

This is a tricky little system that helps pump toxic substances out of cells, or prevent their entry in the first place! Good one, right?

# Your gut and detoxification

Yes, we're back talking about your gut. Bet you never thought about the intestines playing a role in detoxification, right? Well, turn your thinking around, sister!

The gut lining is the first point of contact for most potentially toxic substances as most are consumed orally – medications, food, drink, and the gut acts as a physical barrier to these compounds. You therefore need to ensure that you have a healthy gut, with the lining fully intact, as a compromised mucosal gut wall can more easily allow toxic substances through into your bloodstream.

Another fun fact: your gut bacteria can produce compounds that either promote or inhibit detoxification!

# How to promote complete detoxification

The key is to support all systems and all phases of detoxification. In a nutshell:

1 Nourish your gut.
2 Avoid foods that can damage the gut – sugar, vegetable oils, excess grains, improperly prepared legumes, alcohol and caffeine.
3 Support phase I detoxification. The following nutrients support the P450 enzyme and therefore phase I detoxification:

- Vitamin Bs (riboflavin/B2, niacin/B3, pyridoxine/B6, folate/B9, cobalamin/B12) – the best source of B vitamins is, wait for it … liver! Now go and eat some pâté! If you're vegetarian, savoury/nutritional yeast flakes can also be rich in B vitamins (though not as super as the liver, sorry).
- Glutathione – a good quality whey protein can help to boost glutathione levels. If that's not your cup of tea, increase sulphur-rich foods such as garlic, onions and cruciferous veggies.
- Branched chain amino acids – amino acids are the building blocks of proteins. The best sources are animal proteins – meat, eggs, chicken, fish and dairy. Not juice.

- Flavonoids – these fancy little babies are beneficial plant compounds that can protect against oxidative damage. Rosemary is surprisingly high in flavonoids and beneficial for reducing inflammation. (Note: Grapefruit juice contains flavonoids that inhibit the P450 enzyme. You need to especially avoid grapefruit if you take certain medications, such as statins, as it can reduce the clearance of the drug from your body.)
- Phospholipids from eggs and liver.

4  Support phase II detoxification. Each different aspect of phase II detoxification has different nutritional requirements:

- Sulfation – vitamin A (liver, egg yolks, orange veggies as a precursor to vitamin A), protein, sulfur (garlic, onions, broccoli, cauliflower, cabbage, watercress).
- Glucuronidaton – magnesium and glucuronic acid, which is found in high quantities in kombucha (fermented tea) Smoking and fasting may inhibit glucuronidation.
- Glutathione reactions require vitamins B6 and B12, magnesium and folate. Brassica veggies help with these reactions, so load up on your broccoli, friends!
- Methylation – folate, B12 (both found in liver; folate also found in green, leafy veggies).

5  Consume plenty of antioxidant rich foods and supportive plants.

- Vitamin C (lemons, limes and kiwifruit)
- Carotenes (sweet potato, carrots, pumpkin)
- Vitamin E (egg yolks, liver, nuts and seeds, leafy greens)
- Selenium (brazil nuts)
- Zinc (red meat, shellfish)
- Manganese (seafood, nuts and seeds)
- CoQ10 (animal protein)
- Thiols (garlic, onions, cruciferous veggies)
- Bioflavanoids (fresh fruit and veggies)
- Silmarin (milk thistle, artichoke, turmeric)
- Pycnogenol (supplement).

**6** Avoid things that tax the liver. These are pretty obvious and I'm sure you're onto them, but just in case ...

- Alcohol
- Smoking
- Excess caffeine
- Medications
- Chemicals – from conventional produce, from cleaning products, and from skincare, make-up and perfumes
- Pollution

**7** Drink water, sleep well, and have more fun!

There you have it! Unfortunately, there is a little more to detoxification than a three-day juice cleanse. Sorry! That's not to say you shouldn't do a juice cleanse. I'm not about to tell you to do one either, but if it makes you feel good then go for it! Just don't be fooled into thinking it is going to adequately detoxify your body. As you can see from the above, detoxification requires a little bit of everything all the time! A wide variety of veggies and herbs, a little fruit (especially berries and lemons), adequate protein, plenty of fresh water, healthy fats, minimal stress, good quality sleep and avoidance of environmental toxins is where it's at!

## Recap time

🌿 Having a healthy gut and liver are essential to hormone balance and overall health and wellness.

🌿 When you have a leaky gut, this can create inflammation in the body, affect the nutrients you absorb, and negatively affect all cells and molecules in your body.

🌿 You are more bacteria than human! The bacteria in your gut play a huge role in many aspects of health, so it's important to look after them by eating fresh, whole foods, fermented foods, probiotics and prebiotics, managing stress, avoiding antibiotics (as much as possible), choosing a natural form of birth control, quitting the cigarettes, going easy on the alcohol and not being hyper-hygienic.

🌿 Your poop provides a window to your overall health. Don't be scared to look in the bowl and be a poop detective.

🌿 There's much more to detoxification than going on a juice fast/lemon detox/breatharian cleanse. You need all the things; all the time.

Now that your gut is nice and healthy, let's have a look at what you should be filling it with. On to Chapter 5: Eat well!

# EAT WELL

*Someone has to stand up and say the answer isn't another pill.*
*The answer is spinach.*
– Bill Maher

You'll probably come across many people in your life who will tell you that diet has nothing to do with how you look, feel and perform. I find this very unfortunate and misleading. Yes, I am biased, being a university-trained nutritionist and dietitian. However, if we take a little look at the biochemistry and how our bodies work, and what they are made up of, it's not that hard to see where I am coming from when I say that food can affect every aspect of you.

This chapter is dedicated to going through different food components, why and how they are important, where you can find them, and how much you might need to keep your hormones happy, your body and mind healthy, and your spunk spunky. Please do keep in mind, though, that we don't normally eat foods as individual components, but rather mish-mashed in together when we consume whole foods. As an example, when we eat an apple, we don't just eat carbs. We also eat fibre, vitamins and minerals, and a teeny bit of protein. So try not to get caught up in carbs/fats/proteins. The information in here is merely designed to explain to you why you might want to consume (or avoid) certain foods for happy hormones.

If you're hanging out with a specific hormonal condition, get your highlighter out, because I cover simple and effective food-based strategies for a range of hormonal woes such as amenorrhea, PCOS, hypothyroidism, endometriosis and adrenal fatigue.

# EATING LIKE OUR ANCESTORS

As you read in Chapter 1, I encourage using an ancestral template to guide you in your food choices. Why? Because our ancestors ate real food that was packed full of vitamins, minerals, antioxidants and all of the goodies that your body needs to function at its best. (You'll learn about these goodies and why you need them in this chapter.) Our ancestors ate local food that supported their own community and was not depleted in nutrients from extended travel to get to them. Our ancestors did not waste parts of the animal or plant that they had available for consumption. They knew that these bits and bobs (aka organ meats), were the bee's knees (or livers, do bees have livers?). And, of course, our ancestors did not eat dodgy food-like substances such as vegetable oils, trans fats, processed soy and artificial sweeteners that would wreak havoc on their hormones and overall wellbeing.

Also note that I used the word, template. Emulating how our ancestors ate is a great place to start and take guidance from, but it doesn't necessarily have to be the be-all and end-all. There are certain foods that are often advised to avoid when following a paleo-style diet such as dairy, legumes and grains. We'll chat more about why this is the case, if this is necessary for you, and what to consider if you do choose to eat these foods.

So, you're intrigued by this whole ancestral way of eating, but you don't fancy chowing down on a big hunk of meat for breakfast, lunch and dinner. Good. Nor should you.

To eat like our ancestors, start with plants. As author and journalist Michael Pollon said: 'Eat food. Not too much. Mostly plants.'

Eating a plant-based diet will ensure you get a wide variety of vitamins, minerals, antioxidants and fibre – and fibre is so good for your hormones. It helps with regular elimination, another fancy term for 'pooping'! As I talked about in Chapter 4: Happy gut = happy hormones, once toxic waste products (such as excess oestrogens) are packaged up by the liver, they are transported to the large intestines for excretion via the faeces. If all is running smoothly, these waste products will be eliminated on a regular basis, and hormone balance will be supported.

It's a common myth that ancestral diets are low fibre. In fact, research has shown that most traditional societies ate a load of fibre in the form of veggies, fruit, nuts, seeds and herbs.

Once you've got the plant base, add on your extras: good quality fats and proteins, fermented foods, organ meats and bone broths, and fresh water. Don't stress, we'll talk more about the whys and hows of all this shortly.

The easiest way to follow an ancestral diet in our modern, Twinkie-filled world is to be smart about your shopping. At the supermarket, shop the perimeter where the fresh produce hangs out. All of the junk is on the inside. If you do head into the depths of the grocery store, read the labels! If you can't pronounce something on a label, don't buy it. If there is a whole-food version, opt for that (for example, oranges instead of orange juice). Ask yourself a few questions: Would a five-year-old recognise the ingredient? Would your great-grandmother have eaten it? Would it rot or ferment if left outside? No? Then don't buy it.

Better yet, head to your local farmer's markets. Even better still, grow your own food and swap with your friends. Or if you really want to build the good karma, give some of your grown food away to your neighbour. Gasp! Sharing and connecting! And not in the way that you would do on Facebook. This is real-life stuff, people. Like back in the day when humans spoke face to face and did things for each other just for giggles. Crazy, I know!

Do the best you can, with what you have, right now. In a perfect world, food acquirement would look a little like this: you would milk your own goat up on your prairie, then catch a fish in your stream, gather some berries from the bush out back and harvest some veggies and herbs from the garden, oh and maybe squash some grapes to make some organic wine from your vineyard. We would also have our own unicorns to ride around on from A to B too. The chances of this happening are probably pretty slim. So work with what you've got. What is do-able for you? Don't beat yourself up if everything isn't 100 per cent perfect.

Don't be too hard on yourself either. The poison is in the dose, so don't freak out about enjoying the occasional bowl of ice-cream with warm double-choc brownie. Just make sure it is a once every now and then thing, not an everyday item, because that's when things start to go out of whack. (Don't you love that term? So very 90s!)

## Practise mindful eating

When we practise mindful eating, we can really get in tune with what our body wants and needs. This involves taking time to enjoy your meals and involve all of the senses.

Ideally, take the time to cook your meals from scratch. The process of cooking, with all of the sights and smells, helps to prime the body for optimum digestion. Isn't that cool? The process of digestion starts *before* you actually eat!

Sit down to your meals. Do not eat while standing up. Or driving. Or doing gymnastics. Try to eat in an undistracted manner. That means putting your computer/iPhone/iPad/child where you can't see them. (Obviously joking about the child.)

Right. So you are sitting down to your delicious meal. Now it's time to savour the goodness. The number one thing you can do to improve your digestion, avoid overeating, and enhance nutrient absorption is to chew (see Chapter 4: Happy gut = happy hormones for more on this). There's a reason we have teeth; use them.

Chew each mouthful at least 10–20 times (no, that's not a typo) so all of the lumps and bumps are out. Then put your cutlery down, sit back, swallow, breathe, then go for your next mouthful. Slowing down your mealtimes will give your brain and body time to recognise that you are eating, which means you will be less likely to overeat and, over time, will become more in tune with your signs of hunger and fullness. This means you will no longer need to rely on a calorie counter/dietitian/food fairy to tell you when you need to stop (or start) eating. How nice does that sound? This is what we call our nutrition intuition.

# Whole foods don't have to be expensive

I bet you're thinking, 'There is no way I can afford to eat like this.' Grains and legumes, often omitted with this style of eating, are cheap. But there are certainly ways you can save some coin if you choose not to eat these foods and instead load up on veggies, fruit, fats, animal protein, nuts and seeds. A few bargain hunting tips for you:

- Choose cheaper cuts of meat such as lamb shanks, beef chuck steak, osso bucco, chicken drumsticks, mince … it's all good! As an added bonus, the meat on the bone is healthier for you, as it is rich in glycine (an amino acid), which balances out the methionine-rich muscle meat. While you're at it, why not go in on a cow-share with friends and buy a whole cow/sheep/goat/crocodile. You and your friends can divvy it up between you. It works out much cheaper. Especially if you're eating the organs and making soup stock with the bones.
- Make your own fermented goodies. They are stupidly expensive to buy. Making your own is ridiculously cheap. Check out how to make these in Chapter 9: Recipes.
- Grow your own food and/or buy in-season produce from your local markets. If you only have a supermarket available to you, choose produce that is in season and/or on special. Just make sure it's not old and manky. And, if you can only afford frozen veggies, that's cool too. Often, frozen veggies will have more vitamins and minerals than their freshcounterparts at the supermarket anyway.
- Limit your consumption of Paleo™ foods such as bars, granolas, bliss balls and savoury snacks. Yes, these foods are good for when you're stuck and there is nothing else to eat. They will be free from the harmful ingredients I talk about later in this chapter, but they aren't really health foods.They'll still be full of natural sugars, and they are a sure-fire way to empty your pockets. Marketing at its best, I say.
- If you really need to bulk out your meals with some grains, go for some less problematic ones such as quinoa, rice, amaranth and buckwheat, just make sure you prepare grains and legumes as recommended later in this chapter.

❧ Use the Dirty Dozen and Clean Fifteen list from the Environmental Working Group to help you decide which veggies are best to buy organic (more expensive), and which are okay to buy non-organic. The list looks a little like this table.

| DIRTY DOZEN (buy organic when possible) | CLEAN FIFTEEN (least amount of pesticides; okay to buy non-organic) |
|---|---|
| Apples | Onions |
| Celery | Sweet corn (although |
| Strawberries | often genetically modified) |
| Peaches | Pineapples |
| Spinach | Avocado |
| Nectarines | Asparagus |
| Grapes | Sweet peas |
| Capsicum | Mangoes |
| Potatoes | Eggplant |
| Blueberries | Rockmelon |
| Lettuce | Kiwifruit |
| Kale/collard greens | Cabbage |
| | Watermelon |
| | Sweet potato |
| | Grapefruit |
| | Mushrooms |

# WHY BOTHER WITH ORGANIC?

Eating organic foods means you're avoiding chemicals such as pesticides and fungicides, which are potent endocrine disruptors. These hormone-altering chemicals can wreak havoc on your health in a number of ways, by:

- Increasing production of certain hormones while decreasing production of others.
- Mimicking the action of your naturally produced hormones.
- Transforming one hormone into another.
- Interfering with hormone signalling, so hormones might be made, but the message that they are supposed to send out will not be heard.
- Telling cells to die prematurely (that sounds fun, right?).
- Blocking the absorption and/or utilisation of essential nutrients (we're talking vitamins and minerals here).
- Binding to important hormones, which again means that the hormones will be produced, but won't be able to be used by the body. Essentially, when something is bound, it is unavailable for use.
- Accumulating in organs that produce hormones, thereby disrupting the hormonal process right from the get-go.

If you want to experience beautiful hormonal flow and optimal health, happiness and wellness, it would be worth staying away from these bad boys as much as possible. If you would like to look more into where you can find these endocrine disruptors (and I encourage you to do so, as they lurk in many of your favourite items such as skincare products and make-up), check out the consumer guides on The Environmental Working Group website (ewg.org) and search endocrine disruptors. If you're doing everything else I have suggested in this book and still having issues, this could be the missing link.

# Are grains the foundation of a healthy diet?

Unless you have been hiding under a rock for the last 40 years or so, you have probably been under the impression that healthy whole-grains (such as wheat, rye, barley and oats) should make up the bulk of your daily diet. After all, that is what we are advised by mainstream nutrition guidelines. Eat cereal for breakfast, bread for lunch and pasta for dinner.

But should we really?

I'm not going to tell you not to eat grains. You're a big girl and can make these decisions yourself, but I'd like you to make an informed decision. Here are a few things you should know about this food group.

Grains are super-high in anti-nutrients, which pose a problem for our digestion and absorption of vitamins and minerals. Think: nutrients = good stuff you need in your body. Anti-nutrients = things that will block the good stuff from getting into your body. These anti-nutrients include:

❧ **Phytate/phytic acid:** These bad boys like to bind to important minerals such as calcium, magnesium, iron and zinc, and stop their absorption into the bloodstream. Cheeky buggers! You will absorb more goodness from your food if you ditch the grains, or at least prepare them properly (see below).

❧ **Lectins:** These little proteins can stick to the cells of your intestinal lining, contributing to digestive issues and also affecting the integrity of your gut (see Chapter 4: Happy gut = happy hormones for more info on leaky gut).

❧ **Saponins:** Think soap. These are bitter-tasting molecules that can make your intestinal lining porous (read: they can 'poke holes' in your gut).

❧ **Gluten:** I know what you're thinking. Going gluten-free is just a passing fad. And while I would not suggest switching all of your gluten-filled foods for their gluten-free counterparts (like gluten-free bagels, cakes and biscuits), I would recommend trying 30 days without gluten and just eating fresh, whole foods. I bet you five bucks you'll feel better. Why? Gluten can be damaging to your health in a number of ways, even if you do not have coeliac disease (and if you do, absolutely do not consume any gluten).

- Gluten can cause inflammation in the gut.
- Gliadin, part of gluten, can trigger an immune response and, because it looks very similar to other parts of your body, your immune system can get confused and attack your own cells (this is where autoimmune conditions develop).
- Gluten can activate something called zonulin in your small intestine, which can loosen the tight junctions and contribute to leaky gut.
- Gluten can worsen irritable bowel syndrome.
- Many brain disorders have been implicated with gluten consumption, including schizophrenia and autism.

And did you know that non-coeliac gluten sensitivity is a real thing? Smart science peeps have been studying it for a while. This means you could be gluten intolerant, without having full-blown coeliac disease.

## How to prepare grains for optimal digestion

If you do want to use grains then they need to be prepared properly, which means soaking for between 12 and 24 hours and, (ideally) sprouting.

1  Fill a third of a jar with grains and cover with water and a good splash of an acidic medium (e.g. apple cider vinegar or lemon juice).
2  Cover with a cloth and secure with a rubber band (so flies and fur-babies don't get into it).
3  Soak for 12=24 hours. Rinse and either store in the fridge for up to 5 days, or use for immediate cooking.

OR for extra brownie points, proceed to the sprouting business:

1  After rinsing the grains, invert the jar (cloth still on, obviously), and let drain.
2  Rinse at least twice a day. Sprouts will be ready in 1=4 days = you'll know when you see little sprouts coming out of your grains!
3  Drain and store in the fridge for up to 5 days. They can be used cooked or raw.

# KILOJOULES COUNT ... BUT TRY NOT TO COUNT THEM

It is rare that I see a client who is eating too much food. Often it's the other way around. This makes sense, given what we have been taught about weight loss is to eat less and exercise more.

My job, in terms of weight loss clients, really should be obsolete then, right? If it really were as simple as eating less and exercising more, most of my clients would be Kate Moss-thin. But they aren't. Some have just a little bit of stubborn fat that they would like to lose (for aesthetic reasons), others have more that they need to lose (for health reasons). All are exercising their butts off and not eating enough.

## The problem with eating too few kilojoules

When you have inadequate kilojoules on board to fuel basic bodily functions, those functions will start to dawdle. Your brain will recognise this lack of fuel and signal to the thyroid gland that energy needs to be conserved and to slow everything down.

Your thyroid gland controls all of your metabolic processes and your body temperature. If it slows down production of thyroid hormones, your metabolism will become sluggish, your heart rate will drop and you may struggle to keep warm. What happens when your metabolism slows down, people? You guessed it! Weight loss resistance! If you are, essentially, starving, do you really think your body is going to give up its fat stores easily? Or do you think it is going to hold on to every last morsel to feed your vital organs (and to keep you warm)?

If this wasn't bad enough, your adrenals are probably going to kick into gear to help you survive (especially if you are doing high-intensity exercise and don't have enough carbs in your diet). This means cortisol is going to ramp up and give you a nice little pouch around your tummy that you can't shift, no matter how many crunches you do. (As a side note, crunches are not the best exercise for a lean mid-section anyway.)

Troubles with weight loss are the least of your worries if you are chronically under-eating and over-exercising. This can lead to sex hormone depletion, amenorrhea and fertility issues. (See more about this on my blog and in my e-book *Healing Hypothalamic Amenorrhea*.) But what about the other consequences you might be faced with? Check them out:

- Compromised bone density
- Brain fog and inability to focus
- Decreased performance (in all forms of exercise, including the bedroom, and that's if you had any sex drive to start with)
- Vitamin and mineral deficiency
- Low energy
- Increased risk of heart problems
- Poor memory
- Skin breakouts
- Hair loss
- Cracked and brittle nails.

Not pretty, right? Moral to the story: eat more and eat well! Or exercise less. You choose. I know it might be scary to increase your kilojoules, or eat more of a certain macronutrient, especially after years and years of trying to do the right thing by restricting. But trust that your body will know what to do. When you love your body by feeding it with real, whole, nourishing foods, your body will love you back and find its weight happy spot. So be kind to yourself. If you struggle with this, be sure to try out the strategies on self-love and compassion in Chapters 7: Manage stress and 8: Be kind. They might be hard at first, but they'll pay off in the long run. Promise!

# Working out your kilojoule needs

It's pretty simple to get a rough estimate of how many kilojoules you need on a daily basis. Just plug your own personal values into the appropriate equation for your age below to get your resting metabolic rate (your RMR). This is how many kilojoules you would burn if you lay in bed all day doing nothing.

| AGE (years) | EQUATION |
|---|---|
| 10–18 | {(0.056 x weight in kg) + 2.898} x 1000 |
| 18–30 | {(0.062 x weight in kg) + 2.036} x 1000 |
| 30–60 | {(0.034 x weight in kg) + 3.538} x 1000 |
| >60 | {(0.056 x weight in kg) + 2.898} x 1000 |

Say I weighed 67 kg and I was in the 30–60 age bracket. The minimum kilojoules that I should consume, based on me staying in bed all day, is 5816 (or 1385 calories). Minimum! This is not taking into account any sort of exercise, folks. Then we have to multiply it by an activity factor. So if you:

❧ plan to hang out in bed multiply by 1.2.

❧ are very sedentary, as in you are just going to bum around the house all day, multiply by 1.3.

❧ are slightly less sedentary, perhaps you do a bit of light gardening, multiply by 1.4.

❧ do light activity, such as a stroll around the shops, multiply by 1.5.

❧ do light–moderate activity, such as walking around the shops and carrying bags, multiply by 1.6.

❧ do moderate activity, such as walking regularly, maybe a bit of structured exercise thrown in a few times a week, multiply by 1.7.

🌿 do heavy activity, such as engaging in some intense exercise on most days, multiply by 1.8.

🌿 If you are a ninja, multiply by 2.0!

Let's say I decide that I am going to walk a little each day. My estimated energy requirements then go up to 8723 kilojoules (2077 calories) per day! Just to do a little wandering here and there.

It might be useful to track your daily food and exercise, using an app like My Fitness Pal to get a better picture of whether you need a slap in the face with a juicy steak. But once you get a picture of how much you're eating, put the calorie counters away – especially if you find yourself becoming obsessed. If, on the other hand, you're trying to lose weight and you find that logging your intake helps to keep you on track, then go for it! But again, try not to fixate on it. Kilojoule counting can take up a lot of time that you should be spending doing fun things! (Note: To convert from kilojoules to calories simply divide by 4.2.)

# CARBOHYDRATES

Carbs are so controversial right now, aren't they? There's the low-carb camp, which is swelling in numbers and insists carbs are the devil reincarnated. Then we have the old-school peeps who demand that we need carbs and that they should make up the bulk of our kilojoules. Neither are right, but neither are wrong, either. For some people, a low-carb diet works a treat (we'll go into who a little later); however, for many (especially females), a low-carb diet can spell hormonal disaster.

## What are carbs?

I say carbs, you think bread, pasta, rice, cereal right? But there are plenty of other foods that contain carbs such as legumes, starchy veggies, fruit and even dairy. Lollies and other sugar-containing substances are also sources of carbs (the very simple kind). Check out the list of healthy carb-containing foods later in this chapter (on page 107).

When we eat carb-containing foods, our body breaks them down into glucose. Glucose is a simple sugar that is absorbed from our digestive system into our bloodstream. It is then shuttled into our cells, with the help of insulin, to be used as energy, stored as glycogen in the liver and muscles, or stored as fat.

To the anti-carb crowd, insulin is an evil hormone that we would be better off without because of its fat-storing tendencies. Know this: insulin is an anabolichormone, which means it builds stuff. Yes, fat is one of these things if insulin is released inappropriately (too regularly or too much at one time); however, insulin also helps build other stuff, too, such as your muscles and thyroid hormone, so give it a break.

# How many carbs to eat per day

How many carbs to eat per day depends on what is going on with you right now. The following is a bit of a guide as to how many carbs are best to aim for, given different hormonal problems. (I talk more about eating for specific hormonal problems later in this chapter.)

## Very low-carb diet: 0–30 grams per day

This would also be referred to as a ketogenic diet, meaning your body will start to produce ketones as it burns fat, instead of glucose, for fuel.

This might suit you if you have severe insulin resistance, such as someone with PCOS, pre-diabetes and diabetes (unmedicated). If you are using medication that either increases your insulin or lowers your glucose, you will need more carbs to avoid a hypoglycaemic attack. (Check with your doc on this one.) Some research suggests it might also help with epilepsy and some cancers.

Often, a multivitamin is needed to meet nutritional requirements on a diet such as this (unless you're eating a bucketload of non-starchy veggies, which many people find hard to do). I wouldn't generally recommend a ketogenic diet for optimal health and hormonal balance, for the reasons you can read about below.

## Low-carb diet: 30–75 grams per day

This level also might work for you if you have insulin resistance-related issues such as PCOS and diabetes. Also, if you tend to be quite sedentary in your day-to-day life, not doing much exercise, especially not a lot of intense exercise lasting longer than 15-20 minutes (i.e. you prefer to sit on the couch and watch re-runs of *Sex and the City* than do anything else in your down time). Loads of people do well on this amount of carbs; however, I would not recommend it for anyone with hormonal imbalances unrelated to insulin resistance, as it could place a stress on the adrenals and cause further hormone catastrophe. (A little dramatic, perhaps?)

## Moderate carb diet: 75–150 grams per day

This might suit you if you are quite active and/or stressed on a daily basis. I think this is a sweet spot for most females to be in. If you have amenorrhea or fertility issues unrelated to PCOS, I would head closer to the higher end of this range, if not into the higher carb intake below.

The lower end of this amount of carbs (or somewhere in the lower carb range) might suit you if you have something like fibroids or endometriosis.

## Higher carb diet: 150–300 grams per day

This is still not really mainstream high, but might suit you if you are a ninja, engaged in intense warfare on a daily basis. No, just kidding. But it would suit you if you are crazy active with exercise (60 minutes or more every day, or if you notice that your recovery from workouts has taken a downward turn); or stupidly busy and stressed with work and/or consistently moving throughout your day at ninja-speed. (So you kind of are a ninja, right?) In an ideal world, you wouldn't be exercising like a maniac, or live your day-to-day life under high amounts of stress; however, it is what it is, and we do what we can to support our reality.

This higher level of carbs might also be appropriate for you if you have lost your period and the moderate carb approach is not cutting the mustard (again, not due to PCOS), if you have an under-active thyroid gland, if you are recovering from adrenal fatigue, or if you are pregnant or breastfeeding.

## Some tasty and nutritious carbs to eat

Different carb-containing foods have differing amounts of carbohydrates in them and, for example, 30 g of sweet potato does not equal 30 g of carbohydrates. Check out the following, nutrient-dense carby options to throw into your day.*

- 1 cup mashed potato = 37.4 g
- 1 cup sweet potato = 45 g
- 1 cup parsnip = 35 g
- 1 cup swede = 22 g
- 1 cup beetroot = 17 g
- 1 cup carrot = 13 g
- 1 cup pumpkin =12 g
- 1 cup brown rice = 45 g
- 1 cup basmati rice = 41.5 g
- 1 cup quinoa = 40 g
- 1 medium apple = 25 g
- 1 medium banana = 27 g
- 1 medium pear = 27 g
- 1 cup mango = 25 g
- 1 cup diced pineapple = 21 g
- 1 medium orange = 15 g
- 1 cup grapes = 27 g
- 1 cup papaya = 28 g
- 1 medium peach = 14 g

- 1 cup rockmelon = 13 g
- 1 cup watermelon = 12 g
- 1 cup blueberries = 21 g
- 10 medium strawberries = 10 g
- 1 cup raspberries = 15 g
- 1 plum = 8 g
- 1 kiwifruit = 10 g
- 1 passionfruit = 4 g
- 1 cup cherries = 25 g

\* Measures taken from Cronometer app

# What's wrong with a low-carb diet?

First off, before I get slammed by the low-carbers, let me point out that low-carb diets can be wonderful for some conditions (such as those mentioned previously in the carb guidelines), but this is *generally* for short-term, therapeutic purposes only, not forever.

Now that we have that out of the way, here are a few reasons why you might want to reconsider cutting all carbs out of your diet.

**It messes with your thyroid function:** As you found out in Chapter 2: Hormones working well, your thyroid gland controls your entire body's metabolism – temperature, weight management, poop frequency, menstruation. And most importantly – low thyroid function can slow down *all* other hormone production. Not ideal really.

**It puts a strain on your adrenal glands:** In case you need a refresher on what these little babies do, head back to Chapter 2 and forward to Chapter 7: Manage stress (after reading the in-between bits, of course).

Here's the thing. Our bodies like to have a set level of glucose (sugar) floating around in the blood; not too much and not too little. When levels get too low, if we do not have dietary glucose coming in, glucagon is released from the pancreas, as is cortisol from the adrenal glands, to pull glucose from the liver and the muscles, and build new glucose from proteins. If cortisol levels are chronically elevated as a result of this, it may cause your muscles to be broken down for energy.

**It can lead to reproductive/menstrual issues:** Such as amenorrhea, infertility, and problematic menopause. Building on the previous point, if going too low-carb increases stress hormones, it is going to simultaneously decrease production of sex hormones in the adrenal glands via a process called the pregnenalone steal – where the starting point for sex hormones is stolen away for the production of stress hormones. You can read more about this in Chapter 7: Manage Stress.

Additionally, stress hormones floating around all the time are going to signal to your brain that it is time to fight or flee, which is probably not an ideal time for reproduction. Hormones that are usually released from the brain to tell the ovaries/testes to produce sex hormones and be sexy and fertile will slow down or even cease (been there, done that).

On top of this, carby foods provide building blocks for things called glycoproteins (glucose + protein joined together). Examples of glycoproteins include your pituitary hormones, LH and FSH, and we now know how important they are to our overall lady hormonal health!

**It can lead to under-eating:** If you're following a low-carb, high-fat diet, you will most likely experience greater levels of satiety. You will not be as hungry and probably find you can get by on less food. Great, right?

Maybe great for some, such as those of you who would like to shed a little weight but again, if you are already lean and exercising, have menstrual issues (especially amenorrhea) or you need to gain weight, then you may find yourself in a bit of a rut, as you will not feel like eating the quantities of food your body needs you to eat. (Check back at how many kilojoules you need earlier in this chapter.)

**It's not ideal for some forms of exercise:** If you're doing high-intensity interval training (HIIT), or anything explosive in nature, then this is called glycolytic activity, meaning that you are burning glucose (carbs) for fuel. If you are not obtaining any dietary carbohydrates to provide this fuel, then your body will make it by breaking down your muscles. I see this common pitfall in many people doing CrossFit. If you want to do CrossFit without falling in a hormonal heap, be sure to fuel yourself properly. This means eating some carby goodness.

**It can sometimes impact your sleep:** Now this isn't the case for everyone, but if you are having trouble sleeping try adding some starchy veg with your dinner. Carbohydrates make the amino acid tryptophan more available to the brain. Tryptophan is then converted into serotonin and then into melatonin, which is your sleep hormone.

**It can mess with your gut health:** Remember how back in Chapter 4: Happy Gut = Happy Hormones I talked about prebiotics like resistant starch? These help the beneficial bacteria (probiotics) grow and multiply in number. Great sources of prebiotics come in the form of carbs. Taking probiotics (in food or supplement form) and not eating some form of starch is like getting a new puppy and not giving it any food. Just irresponsible.

These starchy veggies also provide soluble fibre, which can help with elimination of old hormones.

# Sugar: The white devil

A little dramatic, but who doesn't love a little drama every now and then? It's no secret that sugar is far from what you would call a health food. Despite many people saying that sugar is harmless, in actual fact, the opposite is true. How so? The sweet stuff is damaging to your health in a number of ways.

❧ Fructose (the part that makes sugar super-sweet) must be metabolised by the liver. Too much can contribute to conditions such as fatty liver disease, which in turn increases your risk of chronic health conditions such as heart disease, obesity and insulin-resistance (cue PCOS and diabetes). Also remember that we need a well-functioning liver to help keep our hormones happy (see Chapter 4: Happy gut = happy hormones). Fruit in its whole form is fine (as long as you're not going gorging yourself on the stuff), as the fructose is also packaged up with fibre, vitamins and minerals, which slow down the absorbtion of sugars, and help with the metabolism of the fructose, making it less damaging to your system.

❧ Sugar makes your cells 'sticky' and can prematurely make you as wrinkly as a raisin. Sugar consumption produces something called advanced glycation end products (AGEs) – convenient acronym, right? These are free radicals that promote oxidative damage and break down collagen (necessary for skin elasticity and suppleness) leading to more wrinkles, at an earlier age!

❧ Sugar can mess with your hunger and satiety cues, potentially leading to overeating. Fructose heads to the liver to be metabolised into palmitic acid, which then travels to your brain and affects the way leptin (your satiety hormone) acts. Ergo, the message that you are full might fall on deaf ears.

❧ Sugar can lead to yeast overgrowth situations, such as candida, which is going to muck up your gut health, and we now know how important this is for hormones, right?

❧ Sugar can tax your adrenals by causing a release of adrenaline post-consumption. The problem here is that the adrenals are also responsible for producing your lady hormones, but these will be sacrificed to make stress hormones instead, leading to hormonal havoc. When you are on the sugar rollercoaster of peaks and troughs, cortisol will also come into play. When your blood sugar levels get too low (such as when we have a blood sugar crash from consuming too much sugar in one go), cortisol is released. This brings your blood sugar levels back into balance by forcing the body to either mobilise stored glucose (glycogen) or produce more glucose from proteins (often from breaking down muscle). Chronic high levels have the same effect on the adrenals and sex hormones as adrenaline – messing things up!

Now I'm not going to tell you to never eat anything sweet; that's just silly and unrealistic. So here are the natural sweeteners I recommend if you're doing some baking. But just because I am recommending them here doesn't give you licence to gorge on them in any sort of regularity. They are still sweeteners and should be used sparingly:

- blackstrap molasses
- brown rice syrup/rice malt syrup
- coconut sugar/crystals/nectar
- dates
- fruit
- honey (use raw; do not cook as heating honey not only destroys many of the beneficial enzymes and antioxidants, but can cause an inflammatory response in the body)
- maple syrup (NOT maple-flavoured syrup)
- stevia (preferably the green stuff that hasn't been tampered with).

## ARTIFICIAL SWEETENERS ... DON'T EVEN GO THERE

While a little natural sweetener here and there is absolutely fine and nothing to beat yourself up about, I would suggest you draw the line with artificial sweeteners. Why? Because they mess with your hunger and satiety cues, for one. When your tongue tastes something sweet, your brain gets the message to produce hormones to deal with sugar (insulin), and the kilojoules that come along with it. However, when you consume artificial sweeteners, you don't get any kilojoules. This is often touted as the reason why you should choose these bad boys; however, if your body produces hormones to deal with something that never comes, what happens? You have all this insulin floating around with nothing for it to act on.

Like the boy who cried wolf, insulin was primed to push some sugars into your cells, but there was no sugar after all. So it traipses back to where it came from. Eventually, insulin gets tired of being fooled by these fake sugars and refuses to do its job. And here we have insulin resistance. Insulin will still come out (from your pancreas), but your cells will be unresponsive to its actions. The result is high blood sugar and issues related to diabetes and PCOS. Be kind to insulin and your cells. Don't fool it with fake foods.

Also, there is some research suggesting that artificial sweeteners mess with your gut bacteria, and you know by now how important the critters in your gut are!

The artificial sweeteners you should be on the lookout for are:

- acesulfame K ('K' stands for potassium)
- aspartame (think Equal and Nutra-Sweet)
- bleached stevia (such as Truvia)
- sucralose (Splenda)
- tagatose
- saccharin
- most sugar alcohols (those ending in 'ol').

# PROTEIN

When you think of protein, do you automatically think of building muscle? Perhaps you conjure up images of body-builders downing protein shakes and pumping iron in the gym? Protein is so much more than that!

Yes, it is important for building muscle. But it is also important for building everything else in the body: skin, hair, nails and, you guessed it, hormones!

Obtaining good sources of dietary protein is essential. When you eat protein-containing foods, they are broken down by digestive enzymes (called proteases) into amino acids. They are then absorbed across the intestinal lining and into the bloodstream where they can then go and find a new happy home to become building blocks for the proteins in your body.

# How much protein to eat per day

It's rare that I come across a female eating too much protein; usually it's not enough. But if you don't eat enough protein, you'll find yourself pretty hungry most of the time and more likely to reach for the sweet stuff.

Try to have a good whack of protein with every meal, breakfast included, so that it makes up around one-quarter of your plate. Here's a bit more of a guide:

- ❧ meat/poultry = a little over palm size
- ❧ fish = around hand size
- ❧ eggs = at least 2 per meal (1 egg does not a meal make).

# Where should I get my protein from?

Know this: obtaining **good quality** protein is really important for keeping your hormones happy. What do I mean by good quality?

I mean protein obtained from animals that have been raised appropriately and humanely. Opt for organic protein sources where possible if you want to avoid environmental toxins (pesticides, fungicides, antibiotics and the like). If this is not possible, your next best option is free-range (or wild-caught and sustainable for fish), local, and pasture-raised (though pigs and chooks will eat anything, not just grass, and this is fine as long as they are not being fed meat-meal).

The grass-fed element is really important when it comes to beef and lamb. Animals fed grains have a fatty acid composition high in omega 6 rather than omega 3, which is high in grass-fed and finished beef. And no, good quality red meat will not cause cancer, so long as you are eating an abundance of veggies and a little fruit every day.

Also be sure to check out the living conditions of the animal and avoid eating factory-farmed meat. Animals are often treated poorly and end up with more illnesses throughout their life; you can't get health from a sick animal!

Check out my blog on Meat vs Meat at www.theholisticnutritionist.com for more on choosing good quality meat.

# Good sources of protein

The most bioavailable (usable by the body) and complete (containing all essential amino acids) forms of protein come from animal sources. I'm talking about foods such as:

- beef – have a go at the Marvellous Mince recipe on page 226.
- lamb, pork and game meats (such as venison and kangaroo).
- turkey, duck, chicken and their eggs – I love eggs; nature's multivitamin. Fun fact: the yolk of the egg contains thirteen essential nutrients. Eat the yolks! Yes, there is cholesterol, but remember, it's super-important for providing the building blocks of your sex and stress hormones.
- seafood – fish, shellfish (look out for a yummy ceviche recipe on page 224).
- crocodile – have you ever had it? Tastes like chicken! (Yes, I am from Australia!)
- dairy – cow, sheep, goat (why not make some fermented milk kefir, if you tolerate dairy? You'll find a recipe for this good stuff on page 234).

If you're vegetarian, choose some of the following:

- quinoa – always soak this overnight and rinse well before cooking to improve digestibility and remove the bitter taste.
- buckwheat – why not try my Coconut and Buckwheat Pancakes? (See page 214.)
- hempseed.
- chia – there's a ridiculously easy and tasty chia pudding recipe on page 217.
- spirulina.
- good quality, grass-fed, whey protein powder – make sure there are no artificial sweeteners or flavours sneaking in.

Then you can look at food combining to ensure you obtain all of the amino acids to make up complete proteins. Mix the following groups together to get the goods (but remember to prepare grains and legumes properly):

- ❧ legumes + nuts/seeds
- ❧ legumes + grains.

## BEANS, BEANS THE MUSICAL FRUIT

Ever wondered why legumes, such as beans, lentils and chickpeas, make you fart more? It's because of the presence of carbohydrates that are not properly broken down by the digestive system. These undigested carbs then travel to your large intestine where your bacteria have a fermenting feast on them. And what is the result of fermentation? Gas!

Most die-hard paleo followers are anti-legume, mainly because of the presence of anti-nutrients similar to those in grains – phytates, lectins, protease inhibitors (interfering with the ability to break down proteins properly) – and also because our paleo ancestors didn't eat them. (Although there is some evidence to suggest that they actually were part of some ancestral diets, such as the Aboriginals of Australia.)

So should we avoid legumes? If you have any sort of digestive issues or notice that you react poorly when you consume them, then perhaps you should try removing them for 30 days and see how you feel.

On the other hand, legumes have their place in the diet. Not as a staple food, but definitely something to be considered as a semi-regular contributor. (A few times a week should be fine if you tolerate them well.)

Legumes are rich in vitamins and minerals, and they provide wonderful fibre to feed your beneficial bacteria. And they are perfect for meals on Meat-free Mondays and Tight-Arse Tuesdays! The key is to prepare them properly to eliminate those nasty anti-nutrients getting in the way of you benefitting from this food group.

How to prepare the musical fruit:

1 Soak in warm water with a splash of apple cider vinegar for 12-24 hours.
2 Drain and rinse well.
3 Bring to a boil, skimming off any foam as you go.
4 Simmer for 4 hours, or until ready (which could vary, depending on the type of bean used).

# FATS

Fats are super-important for your hormones (and pretty much everything else in your body). Yet we have been led to believe that a low-fat diet is best for everyone except for kiddies under two – those lucky little devils!

Most of us have followed this advice for a long time. I know I did. And where has it got us? We are fatter and sicker than ever before, despite our intake of traditional fats going down.

Ancestral societies not only ate whole, unprocessed, and even saturated fats, but for some, it constituted quite a large proportion of their diets. For example, the Inuit *loved* whale blubber – their diets were apparently up around the 90 per cent fat mark! While I'm not suggesting you aim for this level of fat, or start eating whale blubber, it does demonstrate that perhaps fat isn't the bad dude it has been made out to be.

Let's take a little meander through the world of fats, because what you think of as healthy and unhealthy fats might be a little different to what is actually the case.

# The good

These sources of fat are the ones that you want to include on your plate each and every day. They'll provide you with an abundance of goodness, including anti-oxidants, unique phytochemicals (plant chemicals), fat soluble vitamins, and also a medium in which to absorb these fat soluble vitamins. Remember, whole food sources of fats, the ones that would have been available back in the day are your best choice.

## Olive oil

Pretty much everyone agrees that the Mediterraneans have it sussed when it comes to fat (they are also quite diligent about including an abundance of veggies in their diets). Extra virgin olive oil is a healthy monounsaturated fat (which simply means that there is only one double bond in the chemical structure) that is also rich in phytochemicals and antioxidants.

Always choose a good quality cold-pressed, extra virgin olive oil. Avoid anything that is an olive oil blend – this means it is probably blended with dodgy vegetable oils (see the section on 'heart-healthy' fats later in this chapter). Always read the labels and check that your bottle only contains 100 per cent olive oil.

I like to drizzle good quality olive oil on my salads, like the Roast Veggie and Feta Salad you'll find on page 219.

## Omega 3 fatty acids

These are also known as your essential fatty acids. Your primary omega 3 fatty acids are EPA (eicosapentaenoic acid) and DHA (docohosahexanaoic acid). They make up part of every single cell in your body and ensure that said cells work as they should, which includes ensuring that hormone messages that are sent out actually get heard where they need to be heard, and action is taken to have the desired effect. They also help to cool any inflammation throughout the body, which ensures your cells are firing on all cylinders.

The best sources of omega 3 fatty acids are from animals. (Plant-based sources just aren't as bioavailable, and the conversion to EPA and DHA is long and limited.) Try to include some of the following at least three times a week:

- anchovies
- wild-caught salmon (canned is fine; and if you munch on the skin and bones you're going to also nab yourself some calcium, vitamin D, vitamin A and more! Check out the stupidly simple Salmon Pattie recipe on page 223)
- sardines
- herring
- mackerel
- bluefish
- tuna
- grass-fed and grass finished red meat.
- marine algae such as spirulina is also high in omega 3, if you are adamant about avoiding animal foods.

Some other fun, hormone-friendly facts about the benefits of these fab fatty acids:

- High intake can reduce the severity of symptoms related to endometriosis.
- They can ease menstrual cramps.
- They are especially important for baby's brain and eye development. DHA is key here; it's stored in the hips and thighs so if you're looking to create a mini-human, having a little junk in the trunk is going to be wonderful for nourishing your mini-me, and for keeping your own baby brain at bay.

## Avocado

Like olive oil, the humble avocado is jam-packed with monounsaturated fats, and has many of the same health benefits. Then there are a few other health benefits that this creamy, dreamy fruit can boast about:

- Avocados contain plant sterols, which have anti-oestrogenic activity, thereby preventing excess oestrogen and helping with oestrogen–progesterone balance.
- Avocados nourish our mitochondria (our energy powerhouses), and help our cells to function more effectively and be more responsive to hormonal messages. This means more energy for you, as well as less free radicals floating around that could cause damage to your cells. Less free radicals also means less premature aging and wrinkles. Win!

These perfect little on-the-go fat parcels also contain an abundance of nutrients, and can be enjoyed in a number of ways:

- Add to salads.
- Cut open. Scoop some out. Put in mouth.
- Slice and top with chives, sea salt and a tiny drizzle of balsamic vinegar.
- Cut in half, crack an egg into the spot where the seed was, bake until egg is cooked to your liking.
- Make guacamole and serve with veggie sticks.
- Make a chocolate mousse (see the Chocolate-Avocado Mousse recipe on page 242).
- Add to smoothies for extra creaminess.

## Nuts and seeds

Nuts are a perfect little snack food; they are! Nuts and seeds are a wonderful addition to any and all diets. Some nutty benefits:

- High in anti-inflammatory omega 3 fatty acids (especially walnuts and flaxseeds).
- Contain hormone-regulating properties (see page 124 for seed cycling).
- Great source of fibre and protein.
- Rich source of vitamins and minerals, including magnesium, zinc, calcium, vitamin E, selenium (key for thyroid function) and phosphorus.

But go easy on nuts and seeds. Think back to how our ancestors would have eaten nuts – they wouldn't have had access to bagfuls of shelled nuts. They would have had to gather and shell each little nut themselves. This would have been time consuming and I'm sure they would have got over it pretty quickly, so nuts would likely have been eaten in small quantities. They would not be downing a bunch of baked goods made with nut meals on a daily basis, and I think this is something that we should also heed. Nuts, while wonderful, can be quite high in omega 6 fatty acids (pro-inflammatory), so best not to overdo it.

I like to team nuts and seeds with fruit. The fats in the nuts and seeds help to slow down the absorption of the sugars in the fruit, increasing satiety. Plus the fats help to increase the absorption of fat-soluble vitamins and minerals in the fruit and nuts and seeds.

## Saturated fats

Ahh, saturated fats. They are supposedly the bad guys that are going to kill us. There is so much fear surrounding these fats, which I completely understand, given that it has been jammed into us for so long that we need to avoid them. However, I would like you to entertain the idea that perhaps we got it wrong. Perhaps saturated fat is, in fact, our friend not our foe.

Fats (especially the saturated variety), play many important roles in your body. They:

- keep cell membranes intact, which is extremely important for proper cell (and hormone) functioning.
- are an essential component of sex hormones – without fats you can expect to see hormone depletion–related issues such as amenorrhea, low sex drive and potentially a more troublesome journey into, and through, menopause.
- protect the liver from alcohol and other toxins (and you know how important liver function is to hormonal balance).
- allow us to properly utilise the essential fatty acids such as those obtained from oily fish and grass-fed meat.
- have anti-microbial properties and protect us from bad bacteria in the gut.
- absorb key vitamins and minerals, especially vitamins A, D, E and K, which our diets are often lacking.
- are highly satiating, so you're less likely to overeat when you include adequate amounts. (So even though they contain more kilojoules per gram than protein or carbs, it's highly unlikely you will eat enough to gain weight, so long as you listen to your hunger and satiety cues.)

And these are the saturated fats to love:

- Tropical oils, such as coconut oil and coconut milk.
- Butter. Yep. Your grandma knew it, and so did her grandma, and her grandma …
- Animal fats, such as beef tallow, lard, duck fat and chicken fat.

# SEED CYCLING

Now this may seem crazy to you, but seeds have chemicals in them that can either boost or block the production of certain hormones. So the idea of seed cycling is to incorporate different seeds throughout the month to help strengthen your sex hormones and regulate your menstrual cycle. This is great for anyone with irregular cycles or amenorrhea.

During the first half of your menstrual cycle (follicular phase, days 1–14), oestrogen is dominant. During the second half of your cycle (luteal phase, days 15–28), progesterone is dominant.

I know that those of you with amenorrhea are thinking, 'But I don't have a cycle!' Don't stress; we are going to borrow a cycle from the moon (see below) until yours comes back on board.

Those of you who get your period, albeit irregularly, can follow in the same way, or you can start on Day 1 of your cycle, then switch over to the second lot of seeds 15 days later.

Days 1–14 will coincide with the period of time from the New Moon to the Full Moon (get yourself a moon calendar app to help work out when this is). During this time you eat, per day:

- 1 tablespoon of organic flaxseeds
- 1 tablespoon of organic pumpkin seeds (pepitas)

Days 15–28 will coincide with the period of time from the Full Moon to the New Moon. During this time you eat, per day:

- 1 tablespoon of organic sesame seeds
- 1 tablespoon of organic sunflower seeds

Ideally these seeds should be freshly ground before consumption, but it's not the end of the world if this isn't possible. Add them to your smoothies, salads, yoghurt, porridge, stir-fries or make my delicious Raw Sesame Fudge (see page 240).

# The bad

The following fats are not what I would call real food sources. If we look at this from an ancestral perspective, these fats would not have been available way back when. In fact, vegetable oils and trans fats only came into production in the latter half of the 20th century. They are what I call fandangled foods – your great-grandma wouldn't recognise them, and neither does your body. Buyer beware.

## 'Heart healthy' vegetable oils

Despite the name, you won't find these oils from squishing some broccoli. These are your soybean, sunflower, corn, canola, cottonseed, grapeseed, safflower oil and margarine. (This frankenfood is just one molecule away from plastic – toss it now and replace it with butter.)

These fats are all extracted at high heat and pressure, which leaves them damaged and damaging. They are also treated with harsh chemicals to deodorise and bleach them, and some of these chemicals may remain in the finished product. One such chemical used in the initial stages of making these fats is hexane, a component of gasoline. Gross!

Due to their chemical structure, they are highly susceptible to damage and therefore should never be heated or exposed to light or air. In fact, heating them contorts the fragile fatty acid molecules into trans fats (see the next section). Yet we purchase them in clear, plastic containers and are told to use them as our main cooking oil. Something doesn't add up there.

If veggie oils are transformed into trans fats, how can they be heart healthy?

Veggie oils sneak their way into *many* food products, including (but not limited to):

- Spreads
- Salad dressing
- Alternative milks (think rice, almond and some coconut – check the labels)

- Breakfast cereals and muesli bars
- Crackers and chips
- Roasted nuts
- Dried fruits
- Deep-fried anything
- Store-bought muffins and cakes
- Baby formula!

## Trans fats

Trans is science-code for mutated fat. They can be naturally occurring, as in red meat (where it is called conjugated linoleic acid and is actually good for reducing body fat and helping with asthma, high blood pressure and insulin resistance), but it is the processed ones you need to be wary of as they are strongly correlated with an increased risk of chronic disease, especially heart disease, diabetes and cancer. They will also damage your cells, meaning that your hormonal messages will fall on deaf ears.

They are found in margarine, biscuits, cakes, potato chips ... you get the gist. If you see partially hydrogenated anywhere, throw it as far away as possible.

# How much fat should I have each day?

As delicious as fats are, there's no need to go out and add butter to your morning coffee. Nor should you be guzzling olive oil. (Seriously, don't do this, you'll regret it. Unless you're into the whole 'flush-everything-out-of-my-system-right-now' experience.) No eating nuts by the bag-full either.

Start by adding enough to keep you satiated. Don't go overboard, but don't be stingy, either. As a general guide, you could work with these amounts:

- A drizzle of olive oil/macadamia oil/avocado oil on your salads.
- A couple of teaspoons of butter to your steamed veggies.

- ❧ A tablespoon or two of coconut oil/olive oil/duck fat to your baked veggies when cooking up a big batch.
- ❧ A small handful of nuts as a snack.
- ❧ A quarter or half an avocado with your eggs/salad, or by itself.
- ❧ A little drizzle of some good quality flaxseed oil (kept in the fridge in a dark bottle to avoid light).
- ❧ Regularly include fat-containing whole-foods, such as grass-fed meat, wild-caught oily fish (sardines, salmon, mackerel), and full-fat dairy (if tolerated).

If you're following a low-carb diet (for some therapeutic reason), you will need to make sure you bump up the fats in order to get enough kilojoules. Don't go low-carb *and* low fat – that will leave you in a hormonal heap and moody to boot, for sure.

# DAIRY

Dairy can be a controversial topic in some spheres, especially the paleo/ancestral health one. Is it a yes? A no? A maybe? It depends on the product, and it depends on you and your body.

### Is dairy paleo?

Some traditional tribes do rely on dairy for a large proportion of their diet, such as the Maasai from Africa. And they are some, healthy people. Trust me – I've met them. I've seen them jump (and man can they jump!). For us non-tribal folk, if you tolerate dairy, it can be a healthful food to consume if you choose good quality stuff.

Ideally the milk you choose (whether it is from a goat, sheep or cow) should be unhomogenised (meaning the little fat globules are still intact and easier to digest), and ideally the animal will have been 100 per cent grass-fed. Oh and full fat – none of the low-fat imposter milk. The fat is so important for absorption of nutrients and for nourishing your hormones.

## What about the impact of dairy on hormones?

It is true that cow dairy can have a negative impact on hormones by ramping up oestrogen levels in your body. It can also boost insulin levels, which in itself can create hormone imbalance, by also raising oestrogen levels, as well as encouraging the conversion of oestrogen to testosterone.

Another factor to consider is the protein in dairy. Whey is harmless for most people, but casein can cause issues. Especially the A1 variety (this refers to the genetic breed of cow the milk is coming from), which can be very inflammatory on your body. In New Zealand (and other parts of the world), the dairy cows are of the A2 variety. If you can find A2 milk, you can avoid most of the inflammatory issues.

However, if you suffer from any of the following issues, I would encourage you to remove dairy for at least three months to see if things improve (I bet they will):

- Endometriosis
- PCOS
- Heavy and/or painful periods
- Acne
- PMS
- Fibroids.

## Where can I get my calcium?

If you're going to have dairy, the best sources are yoghurt, kefir (see how to make this on page 234), cheese and full-fat milk. Two to three serves per day is plenty, so you might have some yoghurt or kefir with your brekkie, cheese as a snack, and full-fat milk in a smoothie.

If you're in the non-dairy crowd (or just to mix things up a bit), you can find calcium in other foods:

- Sardines (these are high in calcium and many other nutrients) and salmon with the bone in (canned is great for this, I use it in my Salmon Patties, see page 223)
- Sesame seeds (see the Raw Sesame Fudge recipe on page 240) and almonds
- Dark leafy greens such as collard greens, spinach, mustard greens, beetroot leaves, bok choy, swiss chard, kale, broccoli and cabbage.

# VITAMINS AND MINERALS

Vitamins and minerals belong to the land of 'micronutrients' – they are small but mighty, and absolutely essential to your wellbeing. When you're eating a variety of whole, fresh, unprocessed foods from animal and plant sources, you can easily obtain everything you need to keep your body in tip-top shape.

Now I'm not going to go into what each vitamin and mineral does here, because that could become quite tedious and, really, you can look that kind of thing up on the web. Instead, let's take a look at the best, whole-food sources of micronutrients.

Here are my favourite, (micro)nutrient-dense, super-foods:

**Organ meats:** Liver is amazing when it comes to nutrient density (meaning it is packed with vitamins and minerals). It would have to be my number one super-food for optimal health. And if the thought of liver freaks you out, just think pâté instead. For some reason that completely shifts a lot of people's perspectives on this must-have food. Best to make your own, though, so check out the recipe on page 237 (I'll tempt you by letting you know that it includes brandy and butter; a lot of butter.)

Try not to be stingy when purchasing liver – go for organic. As I talk about in Chapter 4: Happy gut = happy hormones, your liver is your main detoxifier. And while it doesn't *store* toxins, do you really want one that has been stupidly-crazy-busy-and-probably-worn-out trying to get rid of hormones, antibiotics and chemicals that are often used with conventional farming?

Don't limit yourself to just liver, though. Kidneys, brain, thymus gland, bones, marrow (in the bone) are all fabulous for cramming micronutrients into your body. I like the fact that you are utilising the *whole* animal, rather than just the muscle meat. It's a little more respectful of the animal and less wasteful.

It's thought that originally, our ancestors would have gone for the organ meats first and possibly left the muscle meat to last (or even to the dogs), as they knew where to get the most bang for their buck.

**Fermented foods:** I discuss super-foods in fermented form in Chapter 4: Happy gut = happy hormones and also in Chapter 9: Recipes.

**Shellfish:** It pains me that I have a shellfish allergy! Oysters, mussels, clams and prawns are filled with an abundance of vitamins and minerals (especially zinc and selenium) to keep you stocked up on your micros.

**Sea veggies:** Sea vegetables such as dulse, wakame, kelp and nori are wonderful sources of micronutrients, especially iodine, which you need to make thyroid hormones and in turn your lady hormones. (Be mindful though, if you have an autoimmune thyroid condition such as Hashimoto's Thyroiditis, as too much iodine can aggravate the situation.)

**Spirulina:** This natural algae really is special. It's high in protein, B vitamins, antioxidants, essential fatty acids, chlorophyll ( which helps eliminate toxins from the body), iron, and a bunch of other vitamins and minerals. The only problem is it tastes a little like pond scum. Mix it into a smoothie and you're good to go. Or you can bypass the taste by taking it in pill form.

**Eggs:** I've prattled on about eggs already. Hopefully you're into them. Quality matters: go for free range, at the very least. Organic would be better. And no, they will not increase your cholesterol or risk of heart disease.

**Veggies:** The more the merrier, and remember to eat the rainbow, rather than just sticking to dark, leafy greens, which tend to get all the limelight.

# DRINKING AND DRUGS

It's not all about the food, ladies. We need to think about the liquids we flood our bodies with, too. Some, like water, are obviously essential and nourishing for our bodies. Others, such as coffee and alcohol can be enjoyed sans guilt occasionally in the context of an otherwise healthy diet and lifestyle, if one chooses to do so. There are some situations where I would put them in the no-go zone though, so read on to find out if you're in that camp.

## Water

I'm sure you're all thinking, 'Yeah, yeah. I know! Drink more water! Blah blah blah!'

I get it. It's not as sexy as saying, 'Make a super-food smoothie bowl with spirulina, chia seeds, acai berries and hemp seeds.' But it is more important. And a whole lot cheaper!

Water is the fluid in which all life processes occur. Think about that. Life processes – just kind of essential? You can only survive for a few days without water!

Know this: the first sign of dehydration is thirst. So if you're thirsty, your body is already starting to dry up. I like to aim for around 2 litres a day, but this is just a ball-park figure. You may need more (especially if you're in a hot environment, or sweating it up), or you may need less.

The easiest way to gauge if you're drinking enough? Check your pee. It should have a light yellow tinge to it. If it is dark yellow, you're dehydrated. If it is bright yellow, you have probably just peed out the expensive B vitamin supplement you had a couple of hours ago.

# A caveat on coffee

I have a love–hate relationship with coffee. I hate that I love it. I love the taste, the aroma, the routine ... the whole experience. I hate that I sometimes rely on it to give me a little pick-me-up (especially when my baby girl has decided to have a party in the middle of the night and I still need to do adult stuff the following day, like write a book!). I also hate the effect that it has on my hormones.

There is, in fact, a lot of research pointing towards the contrary. Evidence suggests there are many health benefits of enjoying a daily cuppa, such as:

- Improved insulin sensitivity, meaning reduced risk of diabetes and PCOS.
- Reduced risk of liver disease (though too much can indeed put a strain on your liver).
- Improved brain function and better memory – hello, productivity!
- Increased ability to burn fat.
- It's a great source of antioxidants.
- It tastes soooo good – not really a health benefit, but you know it's true!

But not so fast. Coffee (well, mainly the caffeine part of coffee) does have its downsides, especially for hormonal health:

- It increases your body's output of adrenaline and cortisol, your stress hormones. What does this mean? Decreased sex hormone production!
- Caffeine is a stimulant, which can negatively affect your sleep.
- Coffee contains tannins, which act as anti-nutrients, binding up iron and preventing absorption. If you have any sort of iron deficiency, avoid coffee, tea and chocolate when eating iron-rich foods.
- Caffeine can increase anxiety.
- Coffee is a very highly sprayed crop – if you enjoy a daily cup of joe, be sure to make it organic to avoid those endocrine disrupting chemicals and keep your hormones happy.

Pregnancy and breastfeeding should be a time of minimal caffeine (though maybe you can have a little – it really depends on the tolerance of your mini-me, as some does pass through the breast milk). Otherwise, enjoy in moderation.

# A talk about the tipple

Do you drink? Oh my God, you do? Why are you reading this book? You clearly don't care about your health! Kidding. I'm kidding.

I'm not here to tell you not to drink. That would be a bit hypocritical and Grinch-like of me. However, as entrenched as alcohol is in our society, it is still a drug that has adverse health effects, especially on your hormones. There are going to be times when you might decide to overindulge in the booze, and I obviously can't stop you; however, I can make you aware of some of the potential pitfalls of getting on the tipple.

Yes, there are some antioxidants in red wine, but for the most part, alcohol kicks your liver in the guts. Given that the liver is the body's detoxification hub (see Chapter 4: Happy gut = happy hormones), if you give it too much to do, and too many toxins to get rid of, it is eventually going to go on strike, resulting in a build-up of toxins in your body. Not only will you look and feel dreadful, but your whole hormonal system will be thrown out of whack (as it is the liver's job to metabolise hormones), which could take quite a while to fix.

Also, alcohol has quite a large negative impact on your gut microbiome (again, see Chapter 4: Happy gut = happy hormones). It essentially kills the good bugs, which are vital to our health and vivacity.

So, you know it's not a health food. And you're probably going to have a few drinks on the odd occasion anyway.

Ideally, stick with good quality red wine (organic would be best to avoid the nasty hormonal disrupters), and just a couple of glasses at a time of said wine. Next best would be clear spirits, such as vodka, tequila and gin. Then think about what you're mixing it with. Less is more: fresh lime and soda water is always a winning combination.

If you're looking and feeling well then a little alcohol here and there is probably fine. But try to limit it to two glasses maximum per night, and have at least two completely alcohol-free days. And try not to go on massive binge-drinking benders. So unhealthy for your body – and your reputation!

If your hormones are out of whack, if you're feeling less than perky throughout the day, if you're trying to make a baby, have a bub in your tum, or are a breast-feeding mumma, you should definitely steer clear of the grog.

The following alcoholic beverages are best avoided by everyone:

- ❧ **Pre-mixed drinks:** Full of junk, especially sugar and artificial colours. End of story.
- ❧ **Cocktails:** The occasional cocktail isn't going to kill you, but if it is your drink of choice, and you're somewhat of a social butterfly, you're probably going to start to see a build-up of stored joy (body fat) within a relatively short period of time. Cocktails are often loaded with extra sugar syrup, juices and liqueurs.
- ❧ **Beer:** Mainly because it contains gluten. Yes, as you might have realised, I am one of those nut-jobs who thinks most people do better without gluten. In my experience (personal and with clients), people do notice a real difference when they give gluten the boot. Beer is also quite calorically dense and nutrient poor– expect the stored joy to creep on.

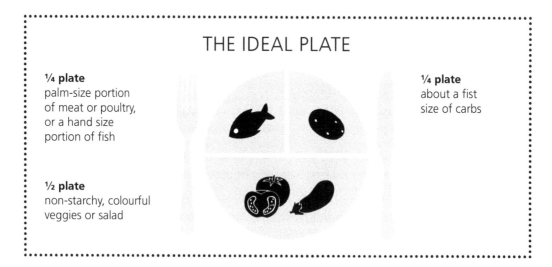

## THE IDEAL PLATE

**¼ plate**
palm-size portion
of meat or poultry,
or a hand size
portion of fish

**¼ plate**
about a fist
size of carbs

**½ plate**
non-starchy, colourful
veggies or salad

So you have a plate in front of you. You want to pile the plate high with goodness, but aren't sure where to start in terms of quantities.

Everyone is different, so your needs will be not be the same as mine. Nevertheless, here is a general idea of somewhere to start, then you can tweak it according to your needs and desires. And please, use a normal-sized plate. No bread-and-butter plate (see the section on kilojoules if you need a refresher as to why), and no jumbo platters. Just a regular dinner plate.

- ¼ of your plate = good quality protein (palm size of meat/poultry; hand size of fish).
- ¼ of your plate = carbs (about a fist size).
- ½ of your plate or more (here is where you can add an extra side plate/bowl) = non-starchy, colourful veggies.
- Add some fat: 1–2 teaspoons at least, unless you have a fatty cut of meat.
- Add some fermented foods: start with 1 teaspoon and build to 1 tablespoon.
- Add some organ meats: a few times a week, especially liver.

This is not set in stone. You might feel better with more fat and less carbs, more carbs and more fat, a change in protein portions, more of everything, less of everything. You can't really go wrong when you start with whole, fresh, unadulterated food and take your time enjoying the experience of eating.

# A MEAL PLAN TO GET YOU STARTED

Please note that while this meal plan (Chapter 9: Recipes) will be a wonderful start for happifying your hormones, if you do suffer from any serious hormone imbalances that do not improve after implementing the strategies in this book (most of the time it takes at least six weeks to see improvements in hormone-related issues), then I highly recommend that you seek out the support of a health practitioner who can create a personalised plan just for you. Invest in yourself – you're worth it!

I like to use a cook-once, eat-twice approach to make life easier. I know you're busy, so you probably don't want to spend all your time cooking meals. Cooking extra at dinner and packing an extra serve for lunch will save you time, money, and ensure you have a healthy option available. So be sure not to forget about putting aside your lunch!

All recipes are:

- ❧ Gluten free – the reason for this is two-fold:
  1 Because it's the trendy thing to do right now. Just kidding. That's not a good reason. The first reason is actually because most people, in my experience, feel a lot better without gluten-containing foods in their diets. And no, this does not mean you should just go and eat all the gluten-free versions of your favourite gluten-filled foods. These are often more highly processed and completely devoid of nutrients. Also know this: there is no such thing as a gluten deficiency. So long as you are including a wide range of whole foods in your diet, you'll be completely fine. You heard it here first. You will not die from avoiding gluten.
  2 Because I have coeliac disease (meaning I really cannot eat gluten) so, perhaps a little selfishly, all of my recipes have been created gluten free. That's just how the (gluten-free) cookie crumbles.
- ❧ Dairy free (or have a dairy-free option).
- ❧ Refined-sugar free.
- ❧ Paleo friendly (grain and legume free).

# 7-DAY HEALTHY EATING MEAL PLAN

|  | BREAKFAST | LUNCH | DINNER | SNACK |
|---|---|---|---|---|
| SUNDAY | Coconut & buckweat pancakes | Asian stir-fry | Slow-cooked lamb shanks | Fruit & nuts |
| MONDAY | Cheesy eggs & greens | Slow-cooked lamb shanks | Salmon patties | Sweet potato brownie |
| TUESDAY | Berries & coconut extraordinaire | Salmon patties | Marvellous mince | Sweet potato brownie |
| WEDNESDAY | Banana omelette | Marvellous mince | Yellow chicken curry | Avocado & chives |
| THURSDAY | Chia pudding | Yellow chicken curry | Healthy fish & chips | Antipasto skewers |
| FRIDAY | Chia pudding | Healthy fish & chips | Roast vegetable salad | Boiled eggs |
| SATURDAY | Vegetable fritters | Roast vegetable salad | Asian stir-fry | Anti-inflammatory super smoothie |

# Some notes on veggies

By now, you are well aware of how important it is to include adequate vegetables in your diet. The more the merrier, I say!

You can include whatever veggies you like; however, I do encourage you to eat the rainbow (a variety of colours) to maximise the nutrient content of your diet and have you feeling on top of the world.

Prepare extra veggies at dinner time to take for lunch the following day. Then you have no excuses not to eat them (you wouldn't throw them out, would you?).

So here's what everyone should be aiming for per meal.

## Non-starchy veggies

Include at least 2 cups per meal (at least 4 cups per day; extra brownie points for adding some with breakfast and/or snacks).

Non-starchy veggies are things like broccoli, kale, capsicum, mushrooms, spinach, silverbeet, cauliflower, cabbage, eggplant, zucchini, green beans, herbs (they are rich in nutrients, too). Anything that's not starchy, really (see below).

A few ideas for how to cook your veg:

- Chop and bake at 170°C for 20 minutes in 1 tablespoon of coconut oil and a sprinkle of sea salt.
- Chop and steam. Serve with sea salt and butter – (this makes everything better and helps you absorb the fat soluble vitamins in the veg).
- Chop and sauté in 1 teaspoon coconut oil, spring onion and/or leek, and a splash of apple cider vinegar.
- Grill (e.g. grilled zucchini, eggplant, capsicum, tomato) with a drizzle of olive oil and some Italian herbs.
- Eat as a salad. Keep the dressing simple (such as lemon and olive oil) or throw some herbs into the mix.

## Starchy veggies

When it comes to starchy veggies, amounts can be a little more variable, depending on what is going on, as this is where you will get most of your carbs from. See the sections on carbs, and eating for specific hormone imbalances, if you need a refresher.

Some ideas for cooking up your carb-fest:

- Chop and roast at 170°C for 40 minutes in 1 tablespoon of coconut oil or olive oil and a sprinkle of sea salt, turning once.
- Chop and steam. Serve with sea salt and butter.
- Boil and mash with butter/coconut oil and sea salt.
- Grate and sauté in 1–2 tablespoons of coconut oil, tossing frequently until soft (like a hash).

### SNACKS TO TICKLE YOUR FANCY

Here is a list of some of my favourite go-to snacks.

- Sweet potato cut into 1–2 cm slices baked in coconut oil and sprinkled with sea salt at 120–150°C for 20 minutes. Turn over then bake for another 20 minutes. These are good hot or cold.
- Nuts dusted with cinnamon and baked in a low temperature oven (around 120°C) for 10–15 minutes or fried in a dry skillet. Keep nut consumption to a minimum – maximum of one handful per day; plain raw nuts are also okay, but not store-bought roasted nuts.
- Hard-boiled egg sprinkled with black pepper or paprika for a flavour boost.
- Sliced raw veggies wrapped in smoked salmon, roasted turkey or bacon (check bacon is gluten, sugar and preservative free).

- Broccoli and/or cauliflower tossed with olive or coconut oil, sea salt and some minced garlic (optional), then roasted in 180°C oven for 20 minutes. Top with pine nuts if desired.
- Guacamole salad: cubed avocado tossed with diced tomatoes, minced red onions and some diced fresh coriander. You could also mash this a little more and have as a guacamole dip with carrot, celery and capsicum sticks.
- Homemade or purchased beef jerky (soy, gluten and sugar free).
- Apple slices or carrot sticks dipped in nut butter.
- Smoked salmon.
- Olives.
- Sliced vegetables dipped in salsa (homemade or sugar and preservative free).
- Kale chips: lightly coat kale leaves in olive oil and placing flat on a lined baking tray. Cook in the oven (around 120°C) for 15–20 minutes until crisp.
- A can of tuna or salmon.
- 1 tablespoon nut butter.
- Fresh, young coconut – water and flesh.
- 1 tablespoon coconut oil.
- 1 handful coconut flakes.
- 1 handful seeds (pepitas, sunflower seeds).
- Hot cacao or cold milkshake made with coconut milk/water, with a little stevia to sweeten.
- Green smoothie (see page 230).
- Chia pudding made with coconut milk and a small handful of blueberries (see page 217).
- Shredded chicken breast.
- 1 tablespoon coconut butter.
- Pâté with carrot and/or celery crudités.
- Cherry tomatoes.
- Bone broth/soup (see page 239).
- Homemade chocolate (e.g. raspberry ripple or fudgy protein bites from I Quit Sugar – head to www.iquitsugar.com).

- Cashew cheese with veggie crudités, roast veggies or off the spoon.
- Prosciutto-wrapped asparagus or rockmelon.
- Guacamole devilled eggs: mash hardboiled egg yolks with avocado and a dash of lemon juice, then stuff into egg whites for a greener take on traditional devilled eggs.
- Sweet banana egg muffins: mash 1 ripe banana and mix with 2 eggs and ½–1 teaspoon cinnamon. Pour into 3–4 muffin cases and top with pumpkin seeds and shredded coconut. Bake at 180°C for 15 minutes or until not wobbly.
- Savoury egg muffins: beat 2 eggs with ½–1 cup of chopped veggies and ½ teaspoon curry powder. Bake at 180°C for 15 minutes or until not wobbly.
- Choc-banana ice-cream: blend 1 frozen banana with 1 teaspoon of cacao powder. If you like, add a small handful of shredded coconut. You can also leave out the cacao and have banana ice-cream.
- 2–4 squares of 85 per cent dark chocolate.
- A few slices of hard cheese.

# I HAVE A HORMONAL IMBALANCE, WHAT SHOULD I EAT?

I promised you some specifics for healing messed-up hormones, so here are my top tips. I can't cover every single detail about healing every hormonal condition (that would be a textbook in itself), so see these guidelines as a good place to start. If you try these strategies and are still really stuck, I strongly suggest working with a health practitioner who can help get your hormones humming to the right tune.

For all hormone conditions, I recommend starting with the essentials – loads of veggies, fermented foods and good quality protein. It's really the fats and carbs, and extra little bits and pieces that need to be tweaked the most.

# Polycystic ovarian syndrome (PCOS)

PCOS is tied in with insulin resistance, so this is the one female hormonal condition I would recommend to limit carbs with, especially the refined variety. Depending on how bad your insulin resistance is, you might need to cut your carbs way back and just eat them post-workout, when your cells are naturally more receptive to glucose without insulin. One cup of starchy veggies or a banana would be a good starting place. You could probably throw in another half a cup of starchy veg or piece of fruit throughout the day and still be in the low-carb range. The supplements chromium and myo-inositol can help with PCOS-associated insulin issues.

If you have PCOS and extra weight to lose (not all PCOS-ers do), then try to stick with three meals a day, being sure to make these good-sized meals so you grab enough kilojoules (see earlier in this chapter), and minimise snacking. You may also benefit from a mini-intermittent fast overnight, whereby you finish eating dinner at 6 pm then don't eat breakfast the next day until 8 or 9 am. See how you go.

I suggest trialling a few months without dairy products, as these can have an insulin-promoting effect, which will further ramp up testosterone levels, leading to those undesirable PCOS symptoms (facial hair, acne, hair falling out).

Finally, increase your intake of omega 3 fatty acids (see the section earlier in this chapter) to combat the pro-inflammatory effects of excess body fat (you can have excess body fat without being overweight) and insulin resistance.

# Adrenal fatigue

Stress causes this hormonal imbalance (go to Chapter 7: Manage stress for more on this). As the name suggests, your adrenal glands have had enough.

We have discussed in this chapter how low-carb diets mess with your adrenals, so if yours are a little tired, be sure to provide your body with regular (around every three hours) carbohydrate-containing meals, so your adrenals can take a much-needed break.

How much carb action? Aim for around 150 g per day as a start, broken up into six meals/snacks, and see how you feel. That works out to be about 1 cup starchy veggies, a large piece of fruit (not berries/kiwifruit), ¼ cup of quinoa or buckwheat groats (uncooked), or ⅓ cup of cooked rice per meal. Adrenal fatigue and hypothalamic amenorrhea are two of the main conditions I believe can benefit from some properly prepared, gluten-free grains and pseudo-grains, if they are well tolerated, digestively speaking, especially if you are sick of gorging on sweet potato.

Avoid refined sugars as this will just put you on a blood-sugar rollercoaster and make matters worse. Also avoid caffeine, as it will just prod the adrenals to do something they're not up to, and make your situation worse.

A couple of other things you might want to throw into the mix with this hormonal issue are vitamin C from food (think lemons, limes, oranges, kiwifruit) and a supplement (around 1000 mg per day), and consider taking adrenal glandular. As the name suggests, this is the adrenal gland of an animal in a pill! You won't taste it, promise!

## Hypothalamic amenorrhea (HA)

For HA you need to do the opposite of everything that caused the hormonal fall-out. We'll talk about the stress and exercise components in Chapter 7: Manage stress and Chapter 8: Be kind, but diet-wise, here's what you need to focus on:

- ❧ Kilojoules. Eat a lot of them. More than your requirements. You need to convince your brain that your body is safe and no longer in a famine. You won't be able to do this in just three meals a day. You'll need to go for five – six meals.
- ❧ Carbs. Again, eat them all! Check back to my quantity recommendations for adrenal fatigue (see above) and use that as a starting point.

❧ Fats and proteins. HA is not about macro breakdowns. It's about eating all the food. All the time. Get some good quality fats and proteins in with each and every meal. The fats, especially, will help you to bump up the much-needed kilojoules.

❧ No caffeine – see page 132 for more on this.

❧ Supplements – acetyl l-carnitine (about 1000 mg/day) can help boost the mitochondria (energy houses) in your ovaries, and vitamin C (also about 1000 mg/day) can help with progesterone production. Magnesium at about 400 mg per day is another great hormone-nourishing supplement. (If you have been diagnosed with Hyperthyroidism perhaps skip the acetyl l-carnitine as it can aggravate the condition.)

❧ Seed cycling – see page 124 to read up on this one (and be sure to try the Raw Sesame Fudge on page 240).

# Hypothyroidism

If your thyroid is under-active, there are a few things that you can do to get your metabolism buzzing again (in addition to following a basic healthy, ancestral-style diet):

❧ Have a daily nourishing thyroid drink of homemade bone broth (see recipe on page 239) with 1 tablespoon each of coconut oil and gelatin, with a good sprinkle of sea salt.

❧ Cook goitrogenic foods that can inhibit the uptake of iodine into the thyroid gland – kale, spinach, silverbeet, broccoli, cauliflower, cabbage … most cruciferous veggies, really. Mix these up with other colourful veggies.

❧ Avoid soy and gluten, which can mess with thyroid function.

❧ Add in some thyroid boosting nutrients:

  • Selenium from 2–3 brazil nuts per day.
  • Iodine from seaweed such as kelp, dulse and wakame (though do be sure to get your iodine levels tested, as too much is just as bad as too little, especially if you have autoimmune thyroiditis).

- Zinc is important for T4 production, and conversion of T4 to T3 (the active hormone). Grab this awesome, fertility-boosting mineral from foods such as oysters, ginger root, lamb, beef, sardines, pecans and brazil nuts.
- Vitamin A, iron and B vitamins. Eat some liver, go on!

❧ Eat carbs. Hopefully you didn't skip the part about low-carb diets mucking up thyroid function. Oh you did? Best you go back then to page 109.

❧ If you need medication, chat to your doctor about going with a desiccated thyroid extract (which provides whole thyroid and all of the hormones you need) instead of levo-thyroxine (which just provides T4, the inactive hormone).

# Endometriosis, fibroids and painful periods

These are all conditions associated with oestrogen dominance, so you want to look at regulating your own hormone production while avoiding environmental sources of oestrogen (xeno-oestrogens). Your best bet, with food, would be to choose organic as much as possible, especially hormone-free meat sources, as the xeno-oestrogens given to livestock concentrate in the fat. If you can't afford organic, choose lean meat (*sans* fat) and add some other good sources of fat (see the section on good fats earlier in this chapter).

Oestrogen dominance can often be caused by too much insulin, triggering a little enzyme called aromatase. Here are the best ways to down-regulate aromatase:

❧ Enjoy foods containing aromatase inhibitors such as oranges, grapes, mushrooms, celery, onion, coriander and fennel.

❧ Lower inflammation in the body by avoiding potentially inflammatory foods such as gluten, dairy, sugar and refined carbs, vegetable oils and trans fats. Alcohol, too, will raise oestrogen levels and mess your hormones around.

❧ Follow a moderate-carb diet (see earlier in this chapter to see what this looks like).

❧ Load up on anti-inflammatory foods – omega-3–rich foods, berries, seeds, garlic, turmeric (see the Anti-inflammatory Summer Smoothie on page 230), pineapple and plenty of colourful veggies.

❧ Revisit the strategies suggested in Chapter 4: Happy gut = happy hormones for optimising gut and liver health. Poor detoxification of oestrogen is a sure-fire path to oestrogen dominance issues. Get these systems in peak form and you're well on your way to feeling better.

❧ Try out some anti-inflammatory herbs such as milk thistle and rosemary; and maybe supplement with borage oil, evening primrose oil and fermented cod liver oil.

❧ Magnesium can be wonderful for reducing period pain, as well as PMS. It's pretty hard to get enough through food alone, so try supplementing with about 400–600 mg per day. Taking it before bed can also help with sleep.

Just as important as what you eat is what you store your food in. Glass, stainless steel and ceramic are your best choices. Ditch the plastics as these are full of xeno-oestrogens. BPA, for one, is a well-known oestrogen disrupter.

# Post-pill amenorrhea

It might come as a shock when you go off the pill and your Aunt Flo is nowhere to be seen. This is quite common. Be patient. As with all of these hormonal fall-outs, it can take some time to bring things back into balance. However, you can help things along with the following dietary strategies:

❧ Support your body's detoxification pathways (see page 87) to help get rid of any excess synthetic hormones that have built up over the years.

❧ Pile your plate (and cup) with the goodies that help the liver get rid of excess oestrogens: whey protein (from grass-fed cows), broccoli (contains a compound referred to as DIM, or diindolylmethane, that helps excrete excess oestrogen), coriander, watercress, turmeric, rosemary, white button mushrooms (cooked), green tea (decaf), dandelion tea.

- Avoid soy, which has plant-based oestrogens and can mimic your body's own oestrogen.
- Go crazy on the super-foods mentioned in this chapter to replenish nutrient stores, and consider short-term supplementation with a good quality multi-vitamin/multi-mineral, and multi-strain probiotic.

# Menopause

If your hormones have left you high and dry (in the lady garden department), if it's been a while since your last period (over twelve months and you don't have hypothalamic amenorrhea), and hot flushes are becoming more regular than you'd like to admit, you might be going through menopause. Low oestrogen is responsible for these lovely symptoms, so try out these tips for helping your body to produce as much oestrogen as it can (there is a limit, though, sorry).

- Avoid caffeine and gluten.
- Eat flaxseeds (see 'Seed cycling' on page 124); these little babies have the ability to boost oestrogen levels. Try a couple of tablespoons per day, added to smoothies, yoghurt or thrown on salads. I also like to sprinkle them on my Banana Omelette (see page 216).
- Enjoy some good quality soy products, such as tempeh and natto. Try to steer clear of the processed forms such as milks, flours, oils and tofu. Menopause is pretty much the only condition I recommend soy for. Otherwise I say there is no joy in soy! Check out The Whole Soy Story by Kaayla T. Daniel for more info.
- Throw some maca into your smoothies. Not only will this help boost oestrogen levels, it has also been shown to increase libido. Woohoo!
- Consider supplementing with vitamin E (up to 400 iu per day), which can help with vaginal dryness, hot flushes and mood swings. Magnesium can help with the not-so-fun side effects of menopause-related low oestrogen. Go for 400–800 mg per day. Pare it back a little if this amount gives you the runs.

# Recap time

- Eating real, whole, fresh foods, like our ancestors would have, is a great way to nourish our hormones and avoid hormonal havoc. How you eat is just as important as what you eat, so be mindful and gentle, darling.
- Grains, legumes and dairy are the grey-area foods – some people do well eating them, while others really do not. A 30–60 day elimination of these foods will give you the answer you're after. If you know you tolerate them, be sure to prepare them properly to avoid digestive distress and get the most out of them.
- Eat enough food if you don't want to look and feel like hell.
- Carbs aren't the devil, and while a low-carb diet can work for some, there are many reasons not to head down this path. On that notes, fats aren't bad for you either! Remember, whole foods contain carbs, fats and proteins. They're all good!
- The best way to optimise your hormones and overall wellness is to load up on real super-foods such as organ meats and fermented foods.
- Different hormonal conditions require different dietary strategies.

Now go forth and nourish yourself!

# TRAIN SMART

*You're in pretty good shape, for the shape you're in.*
– Dr Seuss

So many of my female clients who come knocking on my door with hormonal imbalances are in the position they are largely due to exercising too much. For years, they have been under the impression that they should be doing ***more*** exercise – either upping the intensity, duration or frequency, or sometimes all of these. Yet, more often than not, what they actually need to do is ***less*** exercise. Yes, you read that right ***less*** exercise.

Now don't get me wrong, exercise is absolutely grand for your hormones if you're doing it appropriately. It can help enhance insulin sensitivity, which is beneficial for those of you with PCOS, pre-diabetes, diabetes or obesity. It can also alleviate the symptoms of PMS and reduce period pain (great for anyone with endometriosis). Plus it is a wonderful mood booster, with all of its lovely endorphin-promoting effects.

Some other awesome benefits from exercise include (but are not limited to):

- ❧ Increased muscle tone and strength (super-important for females and no, you are not likely to bulk up if you lift weights; unless you're also on the 'roids, which I don't suggest, for obvious reasons).
- ❧ Reduced risk of injury (unless you're being silly and over-training, which we'll chat about later).

❧ Stress reduction and better sleep.

❧ Enhanced mood (decreased depression and anxiety. In fact, some studies have shown that exercise is more effective than antidepressant medications).

❧ Healthy weight loss and/or maintenance.

❧ Improved self-confidence.

Sounds good, right? I'm guessing I probably didn't need to convince you that exercise is good for you. You're probably thinking, 'Yeah, yeah. I know. Get on with it.' So because you already know that stuff, in this chapter you'll learn when, why and how exercise can be detrimental for your hormone health.

For those of you without a particular hormone imbalance (and just to fill your head with some knowledge bombs), I discuss strength training, high-intensity interval training and cardio – when these might be appropriate and how to implement them into your life. I include some handy training programs for you to try on for size without messing with the hormone balance you have worked so hard to achieve with all of the nourishing foods you're now giving your body. (You're started already, right?)

You'll learn why you need a little booty for happy, healthy hormones.

Finally, just like in Chapter 4: Eat well, you'll find some specific exercise strategies for dealing with a range of hormonal conditions. So get your G-string leotards and leg warmers on, ladies, we're diving in.

# JUST BECAUSE SOME EXERCISE IS GOOD DOESN'T MEAN MORE IS BETTER

The reality is that at the end of every workout you're in worse shape than when you started. (Oh, great!) But with adequate rest, hydration and, of course, fresh, whole foods your body will adapt to cope with these specific stressors that you place on it.

If you're not having rest days and allowing your body to recover; if you're absolutely smashing yourself in every workout as opposed to balancing the yang with the yin; if you're forcing yourself to train when you are already stressed out in other areas of your life, not sleeping well, and really just want to have a nap; if you're training like an athlete (but not eating or resting like one also), then chances are you are heading for breakdown.

It is so incredibly important to listen to your body. It will give you signs that you're pushing things too hard and need to back off. So, what are these signs?

- Increased belly fat and weight gain, despite training like a boss.
- Disrupted menstrual cycle – your periods might become lighter, less regular, or they might pack up and leave altogether.
- Poor recovery – you might be constantly in pain. And if you're thinking, 'No pain, no gain,' then I suggest you give yourself a bit of a slap in the face and be a bit more respectful of your body.
- Sleep issues, such as insomnia.
- Poor bone density – I know this sounds counter-productive as strength training helps with bone density, but if you have exhausted your sex hormones, your bones are going to pay the price.
- Decreased performance – perhaps the amount of weight you can lift is going down, instead of up, despite your hard-core fitness program.
- Irritability and moodiness.

- ❧ Feeling. Just. So. Tired.
- ❧ More frequent illnesses such as coughs and colds.
- ❧ Skin issues, such as dryness, dullness and acne.

Bugger! I'm sure you can agree that these are less-than-appealing signs and symptoms. And if not, if you're still not convinced then I say, 'Good luck to you, beauty. Come back to this book when your head is out of the sand.' I'm not saying this to be mean. I'm saying this as I have been there, with my head deep below sea level, unwilling to pull it out, even though every inch of my body was suffocating. I don't want you to make the same mistakes I did. It's really not pretty and can be a long, painful and frustrating journey back to baseline.

# Why too much exercise can do more harm than good

The reason why too much exercise is problematic is largely as a result of cortisol, your stress hormone. Too much exercise is a stress on the body. And I repeat ('cos it's important to jam into your brain): with a rise in cortisol comes a fall in sex hormones, creating hormone depletion and all of the not-so-lovely side effects mentioned above. The other main reason is that a bucketload of intense exercise will create an energy deficit (if you're exercising like a maniac, I bet your booty you aren't eating a sufficient amount of food to support it), which can be problematic for the reasons we went over in Chapter 5: Eat well.

Also, when you train, you create oxidative stress throughout the body. When you rest, your body has the opportunity to get this under control, and you will come out in better shape than you went in. Conversely, if you never stop, or at least slow down, this oxidative stress can get out of control leading to widespread inflammation and, you guessed it, increased risk of chronic disease, along with the less-than-sexy symptoms of your body struggling to stay afloat.

# Decreasing your exercise – the mental hurdles

I get it. I've been there. I used to be in the extreme-exerciser camp, sometimes doing up to sixteen hours of exercise per week in the form of aerobics, step and weights classes, along with my own extra weight and cardio training. No wonder I became a shell of a woman (physically, mentally and emotionally).

When I finally realised that if I wanted to heal my hormones and restore my fertility I needed to decrease my exercise quite substantially, I faced some mental hurdles. Exercise had been such a large part of my life (both personal and professional). I had always been 'that fit girl with the six-pack abs'. Teaching aerobics was my job! I loved it! It was almost like I needed to change *who* I was. I realise now that this was not the case – there is more to us than what we do, and especially more to us than what we look like!

Some strategies that might help you overcome the mental hurdle of decreasing exercise:

- ❧ **Understand your why:** Why is it that you want to stop over-training? For me, the top motivations were fertility (my hubby and I wanted to start trying to create a mini-human) and bone health (which was pretty average at the time – I didn't want to be in a wheelchair by the age of 40 due to a hip fracture). If you do not have a strong motivator or desire to change then change can and will be difficult. Take some time to sit down and have a think about your reasons (and your priorities). Perhaps write them down and stick them somewhere you can see them on a regular basis.

- ❧ **Start to love and respect yourself:** I know this sounds a little hippy-dippy, but it shouldn't. Unless you love and respect yourself, and see yourself as truly worthy of healing, and of love, regardless of how you look, then you will find making these changes very difficult. In Chapter 8: Be Kind I provide strategies for practising self-love and respect. For the meantime, I want you to start with this:

• Every time you walk past a mirror, look yourself in the eyes and say, 'I love you [insert your name here].' Every time. At first you might experience some negative reactions – you might not believe it. You might laugh. You might cry. Persevere, my friend, as energy follows thought, and if you are constantly thinking negative thoughts then positive change will be stifled.

❧ **Tell your friends and ask for support:** Yes, it is okay to admit that things aren't going swimmingly and you need a little help. Perhaps even schedule in more regular catch-ups with these friends in those times when you would have otherwise gone to the gym. It'll help keep your mind off things, and social interaction is wonderfully healing for the mind and body. Also, when you share what's going on, and what you need to do to get out of your rut, it gives you a source of accountability.

❧ **Crowd out the intense with the not-so-intense:** Slowly (unless you're the all-or-nothing type) switch out your hard-core exercise sessions for more restorative activities such as yoga, tai chi and walking. Change can be scary, so take it easy on yourself and progress as you feel comfortable.

❧ **Acknowledge that you are not your body:** And you are not your score on the WOD board (this is a CrossFit reference, meaning Workout of the Day, which often involves some kind of high-intensity body beat-down). You are a human being. Your friends and family will still love and respect you (possibly even more so) regardless of your body size, composition or activity level. If they don't, they're not really the type of people you want to be associating with anyway, right? Judgy McJudgers!

❧ **Get your priorities right:** Realise that there are more important things in life than having six-pack abs.

❧ **Calm down:** Delve in deep to daily stress management and self-love techniques. (And stay tuned, we'll be hitting this topic pretty hard in the next two chapters.)

# So I might be better off not exercising at all?

No, don't be twistin' my words. I like to say that we need to **move more but exercise less**. Plenty of movement is essential for healthy hormones, and as females we are biologically designed to move our bodies regularly. But this doesn't mean moving at your maximum capacity. It means incorporating a range of movements into your daily life. Movements that you find enjoyable, rather than just doing something as a means to an end (fat burning, muscle building, avoidance of life issues, etc).

Many people believe that it doesn't matter if they sit down all day (on the way to and from work, at work, at home); as long as they throw in one hour of intense exercise at the gym every day then life will be peachy.

Not so much. Haven't you heard that sitting is the new smoking?

So while I am not advocating for excess exercise, I am also definitely not encouraging you to sit on your bum all day doing nothing but watching re-runs of **Gossip Girl**.

If you do have a sedentary job that finds you sitting on your backside for most of the day, try to get up at regular intervals and just **Moooove** for a few minutes. It doesn't have to be anything structured, so don't think too much about it. I like to get people to adopt the Pomodoro Technique, which is actually designed to help people focus and be more productive at work (which it definitely does do, in my experience). This involves setting a timer for 25 minutes, with a 5-minute break at the end. For that 25 minutes, you will focus on getting your work done. When the buzzer goes for your 5-minute break, get up and move your body a little – go for a walk around the office, perhaps outside for a bit of Vitamin D (from sunshine), and Vitamin N (nature, if it's available to you). Try to do this throughout the day and notice how awesome you feel as you snuggle down into bed at night.

# Some intense exercise is great

Both strength training (using weights and your own body as a weight) and high intensity cardio can be wonderful for the body. No surprises there. Just remember that the poison is in the dose, and how much you do (and how often), all depends on your personal situation, as well as how you are feeling at any given time.

Something to get into the habit of doing is a quick daily self-assessment, which can give you a bit of a hint as to what your movement should look like that day: For example whether you should keep it chilled out with some gentle walking (outside preferably) and yoga, or if you can push yourself a little harder with some weights or maybe some cardio activity.

A few questions you might want to ask yourself:

- How did I sleep? How long for and how was the quality?
- When did I last train? (Hint: if you trained this morning, you probably don't need to train again this afternoon.)
- How is my motivation to train today? (This means not telling yourself to harden up if you just feel like poo.)
- How are my energy levels?
- When did I last eat? (This is very individual. Some people train better in a fasting state, others need a little somethin' in their belly.)
- What sort of day/week have I got ahead?
- Am I feeling tight or injured at the moment? (Pushing through injury will quite literally floor you! Don't be foolish.)
- Do I have any glaring hormonal issues that would suffer if I smash myself in the gym such as hypothalamic amenorrhea, infertility and adrenal issues? See later in the chapter for guidelines if you do.

If you go through this list and it reveals that you are, in fact, feeling magnificent and have no hormonal concerns, then get your spandex on, girl, you're off to do a workout. (Sorry – I was born in the 80s!)

# IF YOU'RE KEEN TO DO SOME STRENGTH TRAINING

If you're off to the gym, I strongly encourage you to step away from the machines where you work one single muscle group at a time. (Think leg press, pec dec and that stupid adductor machine that you're using to try to attain a thigh gap – thigh gaps are so 2013). Instead, head towards the free weights, functional equipment and cable machines where you can work multiple muscle groups at once, in a full range of motion, thereby getting more bang for your buck.

Now you might be thinking, 'But I have no idea how to use those dooby dackers (fancy term for dumbbells/cable machines/kettle-bells), and the weights area scares me as it's full of intimidating muscled-up dudes.'

First of all, those dudes are way too concerned with how their own biceps are looking to be focused on what you are doing. And if they are watching what you are doing, it's probably because they are impressed – or they think you're a hottie! There's always the chance that they *are* actually checking you out. Don't let it put you off. Hold your head high, you sexy minx, you.

Second, you could use these guys to your advantage while also stroking their ego a little, and ask them to show you how to use the equipment in question.

Third, why not invest in a couple of sessions with a personal trainer who can show you how to safely use the equipment and possibly even write up a program specifically tailored to your goals.

If you have a little knowledge of using this equipment, a training program for you might look something like this (warm-up and cool-down not included, so please ad lib):

❧ Exercise A1: Squats with a barbell on your back, or kettle-bell at your chest (this is called a goblet squat).
❧ Exercise A2: Push-ups (on knees or toes).

Repeat each movement 8–12 times (depending on how you feel), and complete 2–4 sets of each before moving onto your 'B' block of exercises.

❧ Exercise B1: Lunges with dumbbells in your hands.
❧ Exercise B2: A row using the TRX, or single arm bent-over row using a dumbbell.

Repeat each movement 8–12 times (depending on how you feel), and complete 2–4 sets of each before moving onto your 'C' block of exercises.

❧ Exercise C1: Bicep curl with dumbbells.
❧ Exercise C3: Tricep extension using the cables up high with a bar attachment.

Repeat each movement 8–12 times (depending on how you feel), and complete 2–4 sets of each before moving onto your cool-down.

Note that I haven't added any crunches or specific ab workout in here. This is because when you are using free weights instead of machines, you will be engaging your core muscles with each and every movement that you do. Multi-tasking at its best!

# IF YOU'RE UP FOR SOME CARDIO

If you want to do what's best for your body, steer clear of the treadmills, stair-climbers and cross-trainers.

These machines are just going to provide your body with repetitive motion – same girl, different eyebrows. Over and over again. Not only is this mind-numbingly boring, it's not that great for your body. Your connective tissue, joints, muscles and bones thrive on various loading patterns – i.e. doing different things and moving your body in different directions – out in the wilderness (aka away from the gym). All of this will help to make you a resilient super-woman.

This erraticism in your workouts is also a wonderful anti-ageing tool for your brain so you can be one of those really cool, witty, switched-on old ladies later on in life.

As an added bonus, different loads place different stresses and strains on your skin, so there's a whole anti-wrinkle aspect to this thing, too. So you can look 21 forever more.*

There are a couple of avenues you can head down for some cardiovascular training. You can either go short and high intensity, or long and low-medium intensity. For example, 5/10 on the intensity scale, with 1 being sloth on a couch, and 10 being a 7-year-old child after fairy bread, lollies and red cordial, you should be able to hold a conversation. Test this out by taking one of your friends along for the journey – you can get your exercise and gossip in one go.

The short and high is otherwise known as high-intensity interval training (HIIT) and it really is the new black of exercise. HIIT involves doing your exercise of choice for a short period of time, followed by a rest period. Then you repeat this work–rest routine. The hard should be hard (enough to elevate your heart rate and have you out of breath), and the easy should be really easy (enough to catch your breath). HIIT is wonderful for boosting the metabolism without burning yourself out.

Work intervals between 20–60 seconds with a 1:1 (e.g. 30 seconds work, 30 seconds rest), 1:2 (e.g. 30 seconds work, 60 seconds rest), or even a 1:3 work-to-rest ratio (e.g. 20 seconds work, 60 seconds rest) have been shown to be very effective for fat loss and increasing work capacity.

Many people make the mistake of doing HIIT for too long. If you can do this for an extended period of time (longer than about 20 minutes), then you're either not pushing yourself hard enough in those working periods (if you can hold a conversation, it's too easy), or you are pushing yourself hard enough and just not listening to your body when it is saying, 'Enough already, woman! I'm cooked!'

*This may be an exaggeration, so don't hold me to it.

# TABATA TRAINING

One of my favourite styles of HIIT training is Tabata training. This involves just four minutes of interval training, and has been shown to be as effective (if not more so) than 30 minutes running on a treadmill.

Four minutes versus 30 minutes for the same results … Hmmm, I know which one I would prefer!

You do eight rounds of exercise. Each round is 20 seconds of work, followed by 10 seconds of rest. Total = four minutes. Winning!

To give you a bit of an idea, you could do something like this (and you don't need to be in a gym or have any equipment other than your gorgeous self to do this):

- Squats for 20 seconds, rest for 10 seconds.
- Push-ups for 20 seconds (do these on your knees, if you want), rest for 10 seconds.

Repeat these two intervals four times for a total of eight rounds, for four minutes. You should be feeling well shagged by the end of it. The trick is to go as hard and as fast as you can during those working periods. If you complete the eight rounds and feel like you could go again, that's a sign that you could have pushed a bit harder.

If, like me, you need more variety to keep you sane (I'm a Gemini – slightly crazy), you might do a combo of four difference exercises, such as:

- Squats
- Push-ups
- Lunges
- Mountain climber (in plank position and doing a 'running' motion while you're down there. If you're puzzled by this, head over to YouTube and search 'mountain climber').

You repeat this circuit twice.

Using these total body exercises helps create a pumping effect, which serves as a kind of detoxification for your cells, helping to drive waste products out, and nutrients in (i.e. out with the bad and in with the good).

If all is looking fine and dandy in your life and you're feeling sprightly, I might suggest doing this style of training two or three times a week. And if you're in the camp of needing a little more exercise in your life, there really is no excuse not to – it's only four minutes, after all! If you've got kids, why not do it with them?

# What about the long and slow style of cardio?

This is the style of movement that we, as females, are biologically designed to do. Think hunter-gatherer. Men hunt (intermittent sprinting to hunt down something for dinner), women gather (long slow hiking activity to collect the other bits and pieces that will make up the meal). I'm not trying to be sexist here. Just looking at things as they were, so don't get all Germaine Greer on me.

You need to be aware of your intensity barometer with this style of exercise, as I can bet your booty, most of you will go too hard, which defeats the purpose.

So you want to be working at about a 5/10 – at this level you should be able to hold a consistent gossip session with your bestie. Or you could sing. Or both. You choose.

This long and slow stuff helps to boost your mitochondrial density. Your mitochondria are your energy powerhouses living inside your cells. So, if you have *more* mitochondria, you can expect to have *more* energy. Now I don't see many people telling me that they don't want or need any more energy. The more the better, right?

Long and slow cardio is also very restorative on the body. It's a nice break from the hard-core stuff you might be doing. You might consider doing this a couple of times per week. If you're just starting out in this whole exercise thing, do this style four times per week and skip the high intensity biz until your body is more comfortable with, and less likely to be injured by, regular activity.

Some examples include 30–60 minutes of:

- Dancing
- Brisk walking
- Yoga – vinyasa flow (although sometimes this can be kicked into high gear, so just be aware of this)
- Slow jogging
- Hiking
- Swimming
- Cycling
- Low intensity circuit training
- Any activity where you have continuous movement, really.

# I'VE GOT SOME WEIGHT TO LOSE, HOW SHOULD I EXERCISE?

To shift the weight, base everything more around the long and slow intensity to start – for four to six weeks – then start to introduce high intensity a few times a week. You should also try to get some weights in there somewhere.

Your program might look a little like this:

- Sunday: Long and slow cardio
- Monday: Weights
- Tuesday: Rest day
- Wednesday: Long and slow cardio
- Thursday: Weights
- Friday: Long and slow cardio
- Saturday: Rest day

After four to six weeks, tack on a Tabata (see page 160) at the end of your weights sessions. Feel free to do something gentle (such as walking or hatha/yin yoga) on one or two of the rest days if you are feeling sprightly.

If you're new to exercising up to it, do yourself a favour and get a couple of sessions with a personal trainer, just to make sure you're doing what is going to get you the fastest results and, more importantly, keep you injury free.

# YOU NEED A LITTLE BOOTY FOR HEALTHY HORMONES

I'm not discounting that some of you may have some fat to lose, but let's be realistic about things. I know a lot of you are probably of the mindset 'the less, the better', but I have some food for thought for you: adequate body fat is actually really important for healthy hormones. Especially for healthy hormones and fertility!

*Femininity for me means happiness and freedom ... freedom of being who you are in whatever shape or size you come in.*
– Kate Winslet

How so? Let me tell you a little story ...

I used to have a bit of a body-fat phobia. Although at 13 per cent body fat, I didn't really have that much to worry about from what other people would think.

Problem was, this lack of body fat was contributing to my amenorrhea, lack of ovulation, and subsequent infertility. I looked healthy (not really, in hindsight), but my reproductive dysfunction indicated otherwise. I knew I had to get this sorted, and fast, as my partner and I were trying to conceive.

I consulted a few of my health practitioner friends. They all suggested that maybe putting on some body fat might help kick things back into gear. As a group fitness instructor who was paid to stand up in front of others in skimpy lycra, this was the last thing I wanted to do. Being the stubborn person I was, I needed justification as to why, and how, fat would help to restore my fertility. Cue leptin.

Leptin is one of the more recently discovered hormones and is often referred to as the anti-obesity hormone. In fact, the word leptin is derived from the Greek term leptos meaning thin. This little hormone, which is produced predominantly in adipocytes (fat cells), conveys information to the brain about the amount of energy available in the body. Leptin levels rise with increasing food intake, telling the brain, 'All is well. We have sufficient nutrients to do our thang. And they fall in times of food deprivation, telling the brain, 'Things aren't so good. Looks like we're in a famine and need to shut off non-vital functions.' Unfortunately, reproduction is one of those non-vital functions. We do not need to reproduce in order to survive. Simple as that.

But really, it's not as simple as that. We now know that leptin acts as more than just an energy thermostat. Indeed there are over 19 000 papers that have been published on leptin (no, I have not read them all, sorry), showing that leptin has various physiological roles.

But back to the case in point. Aside from signalling energy sufficiency to my brain, how would body fat and as a by-product of increased body fat, leptin, help me to recover from hypothalamic amenorrhea and restore my fertility?

Remember back in Chapter 2: Hormones working well we spoke about what a healthy menstrual cycle looks like? And we spoke about the role of FSH and LH? (Flick back to page 37 if you need a refresher.) FSH and LH (also called gonadotropins) are pretty important. Without them, your sex organs would not receive the message to produce your sex hormones, or to ovulate, or to menstruate. But we are missing an important step. FSH and LH need a little encouragement too, and this comes in the form of another hormone – gonadotopin releasing hormone (GnRH), which is released by the hypothalamus. Quick recap – GnRH stimulates the release of FSH and LH, which promote ovarian function and a healthy menstrual cycle.

Now here's the kicker. Leptin has been found to play a regulatory role in GnRH secretion and hence, overall reproductive function. Whether this is a direct or indirect role remains to be discovered. However, what we do know is that women with amenorrhea tend to have lower leptin levels than women with healthy ovulatory cycles as a result of low body fat and/or increased physical activity and/or insufficient food. These low levels of leptin then contribute to alterations in GnRH secretion, as evidenced by disruptions to LH secretion.

Now I know what you're thinking, what happens if we just give someone leptin? Will that get things back on track? In one study a small number of women with hypothalamic amenorrhea were treated with leptin over a period of three months and found that the treatment did restore menstruation, ovulation and hence, fertility.In another study, leptin therapy resulted in 70 per cent of women getting their period back, and 60 per cent of these women also ovulated.

Woohoo! Let's all go and get us some leptin to inject – or we could just eat more, exercise less and embrace our booty!

This is probably a better strategy, as I think you'll be pretty hard-pressed to find some injectable leptin.

After two years of being in denial about the importance of body fat and desperately holding on to my washboard stomach (which I had thought was my defining feature), I succumbed. I ate more. I exercised less. I put on (quite) a bit of body fat. And I realised that my friends and family probably loved me for more than just my body.

I put on weight. That was the goal, after all. One other lovely effect was that my period returned. Hurrah! It just goes to show that with a little dedication and a (pretty big) mental shift, beautiful things can happen.

Your period is a luxury, not a right, and definitely not an inconvenience! If your lady holiday is MIA, see it as the canary in the coalmine and do something about it before things really go south. Stop trying to reach some warped perception of the ideal body and start embracing your natural feminine curves. And remember, you are so much more than what you look like. Be kind to yourself for once.

# I HAVE A HORMONAL IMBALANCE, HOW SHOULD I EXERCISE?

Great question! It depends on what kind of hormonal imbalance you have, so let's have a look at a few examples that require exercise tweaking. Note that not all of the hormonal conditions mentioned in Chapter 5: Eat well are covered here; if you have one of these hormonal conditions, you should be fine to exercise as you wish – not too little, not too much, and as much variety as possible.

## Hypothalamic amenorrhea (HA)

Just in case you've forgotten or skipped Chapter 3: Hormones Going Haywire, HA refers to a missing period due to not enough food and/or too much exercise and/or not enough body fat and/or too much stress.

I start with this one, as this is my specialty, having been-there-done-that myself.

To reverse HA and get your period back, you need to get your energy availability up (by burning less kilojoules), your stress levels down, and your brain back in a happy and relaxed state.

When you have HA, you need to avoid exercises that are stressful and/or taxing on the body, including:

❧ Running.
❧ High-impact aerobics classes (think Body Attack, Body Step, Body Combat – I used to do these every day).
❧ Long weights sessions (i.e. longer than 30 minutes).
❧ Most high-intensity interval training (HIIT) such as CrossFit or F45 cardio classes. The exception, in some cases, is Tabata training, which you read about previously.
❧ Medium-high intensity cardio activity that lasts longer than 15–20 minutes.

*I believe that the Good Lord gave us a finite number of heartbeats and I'm damned if I'm going to use up mine running up and down a street.*
– Neil Armstrong

I know this sounds like a big change, and it is. This does not mean you will never be able to participate in these activities ever again. It just means that they are not the best choice for you right now.

Instead, choose activities that restore rather than deplete the body ***and*** the mind. Movement that will not raise cortisol levels through the roof. Make choices that calm you down as opposed to ramping you up. Some examples include:

- Yoga – I cannot speak highly enough of including yoga in the healing process for HA (and any healing process, for that matter). Not only is it wonderful for balancing hormones and keeping you physically strong and supple, it is absolutely amazing for helping you to appreciate your body's ability, rather than it's aesthetics. Yoga helps you to escape your crazy female brain (you know what I'm talking about). Try styles such as vinyasa, yin and hatha, as opposed to bikram or ashtanga. My favourite online yoga resource, for those of you who can't make it to classes, is YogaGlo. In fact, everyone can benefit from yoga and should add it into their lives to reap the hormonal rewards. Resist the urge to run out before the final relaxation (Chavasana) because you think it's boring. If you experience this urge, or get fidgety during this final resting pose, then you probably need to stay there for longer than everyone else!
- Walking (preferably in nature). Again, this is good for everyone!
- Short weights sessions (less than 30 minutes and focused on whole body, functional movements). When I first started my healing journey, I was simply doing 10 minutes of heavy lifting twice a week – it kept me feeling strong without stressing out my body.
- Short bursts of cardio one or two times per week, such as Tabata training
- Gentle swimming – less than 30 minutes.
- Vibration platform – spending 10–20 minutes on a vibration platform two or three times a week can help with strengthening bones. Hopefully you have access to one!

❧ Sex/orgasm – I included orgasm as opposed to just sex in case you don't have a partner. Why orgasm? This is a powerful stress reliever and helps to encourage blood flow to your nether regions!

Also consider this: only exercise if and when you feel you have the energy to do so. Do not use exercise as a way of giving yourself more energy. That's what sleep and food are for!

A training week for you might look like this:

❧ Monday: Weights  (30 minutes maximum)
❧ Tuesday: Yoga
❧ Wednesday: Tabata
❧ Thursday: Yoga
❧ Friday: Weights (30 minutes maximum)
❧ Saturday: Long, slow walk in nature
❧ Sunday: Rest

Even though you need to keep exercise to a minimum, movement is still important for physical and mental health. Feel free to add in daily, slow walks to this program. Also acknowledge that this might in fact be too much for you. If you are doing everything in your power to get your period back (by eating more and managing stress) and it is still MIA with this level of exercise, take it as a sign that you need to pull back even further. Perhaps all the way back to just slow, leisurely walking.

Once your period comes out of hiding, then you can gradually add in small amounts of exercise and monitor how it affects you. If your monthlies disappear again, you've pushed too hard and need to take a step back. It can be a tedious process, but eventually you will find your exercise sweet spot that won't harm your hormones.

# PCOS, pre-diabetes, diabetes and obesity

As you have learned (see Chapter 3: Hormones going haywire for a refresher), a key marker of these conditions is insulin resistance. If you can improve insulin sensitivity (your cell's responsiveness to insulin), then you can manage the symptoms of these conditions more effectively, as improving insulin sensitivity means your pancreas needs to produce less insulin to deal with any given amount of glucose (from carbs). This also means less of your oestrogen will be converted into testosterone (ergo, less man-like symptoms associated with PCOS, which I'm sure you will agree is desirable). It also means that your body will be better able to tap into fat-burning mode.

With that in mind, what's one of the best ways to improve insulin sensitivity? Resistance training aka lifting weights! If you have PCOS (or any insulin resistance issues, for that matter, such as diabetes), start pumping some iron, baby.

How often? Two or three times a week would be super, but if you're new to the whole thing, start off easy and see how you go. You might find you're a little sore the first few times you train. Don't worry, this gets better, and more bearable. The weights program provided earlier in the chapter would be a good start.

Handy reminder for all my lovely PCOS-ers: keep the majority of your carb intake in that post-workout window (within three hours of working out), as your cells will be extra sensitive to glucose and be able to suck it up from the blood via a mechanism called non-insulin-mediated glucose transport. In English, you don't require insulin to get glucose into your cells where it is needed (or at least you won't need as *much* as if you were to carb-up while sitting on your bum all day (which I do not recommend at all).

# Adrenal conditions

This is a tricky one. Depending on how far down the rabbit hole of adrenal burnout (from excess stress) you are, you may need to pull right back on the exercise. If you struggle to drag yourself out of bed in the morning, need coffee to act like a normal human, and then want to crawl under your desk for a nap by 3 pm, you probably need a well-earned rest.

If this is you, I would recommend sticking to just walking and yoga (preferably just hatha and yin styles, rather than bikram or ashtanga. Gentle vinyasa might be okay, too), until you come back to the land of the living.

Once you start to feel a little more functional, you can dabble with adding in weights and a *tiny* amount of cardio – keep them short and low intensity to start. It is really key to listen to your body with this one to avoid putting yourself back at square one, or worse off than when you started. If your body is telling you that it is tired, that it is in pain, or that your recovery is bad, then back off until you hear it say, 'Okay, babe – let's try again. This time a little more gently, please.'

A training week for you might look like this:

- Monday: Yoga
- Tuesday: Walk
- Wednesday: Walk
- Thursday: Yoga
- Friday: Walk
- Saturday: Yoga
- Sunday (Rest – get outdoors and do something fun with your loved ones)

The more you can get outside for your exercise with adrenal fatigue, the better, as this will help to regulate cortisol and your circadian rhythms.

# Pregnancy/breastfeeding

There is no doubt that exercise during pregnancy can be a wonderful thing – for you and for bubs. And when you're breastfeeding a little human, doing some movement is almost essential to keep you sane (and get you out of the house, hopefully).

In saying that, you need to be mindful of how your body is feeling, and respond accordingly. In most cases, the rule goes like this: whatever your level of exercise prior to falling pregnant was, you can continue exercising at this level. If you have any complications, obviously things will be different and you should always get the go-ahead from your primary health provider.

There are some things you won't be able to do when pregnant, though:

- Deep yoga twists (always tell your instructor if you are pregnant, so you can get some extra TLC).
- Core work (e.g. crunches).
- Later on when your belly is big, avoid lying on your back as this places pressure on your vena cava, which can limit blood flow to both you and bubs.
- Intense exercise in heated environments – you want to keep your core body temperature down.

And for when you are breastfeeding and pregnant:

- Ensure adequate hydration.
- Ensure you have more than enough food on board before and after – you're nourishing a human being, after all!
- Listen to your body!

# A FEW MORE TIPS ON EXERCISING FOR HEALTHY HORMONES

1  **Make it fun.** Hitting the treadmill for an hour is boring! I wouldn't blame you for not keeping this up long-term. Find something that you actually enjoy doing, as this will help keep you on track and will minimise stress hormone output. Result = happy hormones and happy you! Add another fun factor by teaming up with a friend or two so it can double as a little social get-together. And don't be scared to think outside the box – what about something like rock-climbing, dancing, trampolining, trapeze or go old-school with some roller-blading. The options are endless – exercise doesn't have to be (and shouldn't be, in my opinion) limited to the gym. Quick fun fact: sex is an awesome exercise choice as not only is it moving and utilising many of your body's muscles, it's also a wonderful stress reliever and hugely beneficial for your hormones, especially if you have any reproductive hormone–related issues.

2  **Variety is key.** Try not to do the same thing day-in, day-out. Again, boring! Plus it doesn't provide your body with enough stimulus to make adaptations and get stronger, fitter and healthier.

3  **Incorporate rest days.** I think I have probably got my point across about this one, but if you really want to get the most out of your exercise without compromising your hormones, you need to schedule in some chill-out time. This doesn't necessarily have to mean sitting on the couch all day (though it could if that's what you feel like on the odd occasion). A rest day could include some gentle yoga, a leisurely walk outside with friends, a frolic in the ocean, or rolling around with your kids at home.

4  **Did I mention yoga?** Seriously, bending yourself into a pretzel does wonderful things for your hormones, your physical fitness, and your mental, emotional and spiritual health. If you can't get yourself into a pretzel, don't worry, it's not really about that. Many women I know avoid yoga because they aren't good at it, or they can't do flying pigeon pose straightaway. Or they don't look the part. If that's you, then I encourage

you to take a deep breath, open your mouth and sigh out those insecurities. Yoga is about the journey, not the destination. It's not about being bendy, or skinny, or eating kale. It's about showing up, listening to what your body wants and needs in that very moment, and responding with love and compassion.

## Recap time

- ❧ **Train smarter, not necessarily harder or longer. More is not always better. A lot of the time, with exercise, less can be more.**
- ❧ **Too much exercise stresses the body and depletes sex hormones.**
- ❧ **We need to move our bodies on a regular basis, in a variety of ways, to reap the benefits of exercise and optimise our hormonal health. Think a little of everything – weights, cardio, yoga.**
- ❧ **Make it fun! You'll be more likely to stick to it, and be in a better frame of mind, which will boost the reward.**
- ❧ **Remember that some body fat is required for healthy hormone function.**
- ❧ **If you're dealing with a specific hormonal condition (and you want to get things healed), you can't just exercise willy-nilly. Go back and read the suggestions in this chapter.**

Time to deal with our crazy female brains now ... the next chapter is all about managing stress.

# MANAGE STRESS

*We think too much and feel too little.*
– Charlie Chaplin

Looking back, I would have to say that stress was probably the number one factor contributing to my hormone issues. At the point when my period went MIA and I subsequently became infertile, I was teaching at least six aerobics classes per week, studying full time at university and part time online, working part-time in PR and planning a wedding. Gotta love hindsight, right?

If your diet is perfect and you're still experiencing symptoms of hormonal imbalance, or feel that something is not quite right, stress is likely the culprit.

I know that stress is likely to be the last thing that you will want to changebut let me tell you, if you start with stress management, you'll be putting yourself ahead of the game, my friend.

Stress management isn't sexy. It's not like the latest super-food berry or green powder that you can just throw in your morning smoothie and Bob's your uncle. It takes a little more time and dedication than that. But the best part? It's almost always free!

In this chapter, you'll learn what I mean by stress management, how stress can have a disastrous impact on your hormones, how to tell if you have been burning the candle at both ends for too long (and what to do about it), as well as a bucketload of fun ideas to help you keep your stress levels in check on a daily basis.

So, beauty, pour yourself a cuppa and kick back in your favourite chair. It's time to embrace chill-out time.

# WHAT DO I MEAN BY STRESS MANAGEMENT?

Stress management involves going against what society deems to be important. It involves disconnecting (from technology) and reconnecting (to yourself, to nature and to real life people. Fancy that!). It involves forgetting your to-do list for a moment. It involves slowing down and taking a moment for you. It involves showing yourself a little love (which I have devoted a whole chapter to – Chapter 8: Be kind).

When I discuss the importance of managing stress with clients, I can almost see their eyes glaze over. It is such an inherent part of our lives these days that we just accept it. Despite it wreaking havoc on our health, it seems to be the one factor we are least willing to address.

I get it, though, as I have been there. I used to be that chick who wore stress as a badge of honour. I thought that me being stressed was a sign that I was busy, which was a sign that I was successful. Ridiculous, I know, but I am sure many of you can relate.

I see it so much in society today. If we don't push it on ourselves, it is pushed on us by others. Especially as women, we are expected (by others, and ourselves), to be able to do everything, all the time. And it can come from every which way.

# HOW STRESS AFFECTS YOUR HORMONES

Let's first talk about what happens when we are stressed. In point form, shall we?

- You are faced by a big grizzly bear who is ready to eat you.
- You think, 'Hell! I've got two options: I could attempt to fight this grizzly; or I could run for my life. Yes, I'll run – backwards 'cos apparently that's how to do it with bears.'
- Your brain registers your choice and releases a hormone called corticotopin-releasing factor (CRF) from the hypothalamus.
- The release of CRF causes your pituitary gland to secrete adrenocorticotropic releasing hormone (ACTH), which triggers the adrenal glands to secrete cortisol, adrenaline and noradrenaline. (Remember, these are your stress hormones.)
- Cortisol increases your heart rate, elevates your blood pressure, mobilises glucose and boosts your energy to help you get away from the grizzly. Cortisol also suppresses non-essential functions, or those that are not needed in a fight-or-flight situation, such as reproductive function.

So this is all good and well when faced with a grizzly bear – it's what we have the stress response for – but how often does that occur? Not often, I hope! However, what we are faced with these days is chronic stress, which triggers the same response, just an extended version of it. And this is what causes issues with hormones.

# Cue the pregnenolone steal

Here's something you might not know. Cortisol can be a bit of a slimy thief. You see, your sex hormones and your stress hormones have the same precursor (starting material), known as pregnenalone. Side note: pregnenalone needs cholesterol in order to be produced. So, eat your fats!

If your body senses that you are in danger (and this could be due to your response to something insignificant, such as heavy traffic), stress-hormone production will be prioritised at the expense of sex hormones, with pregnenolone being shuttled towards cortisol, as opposed to oestrogen. Thief! Hence you will end up being deprived of sex hormones and all of the lovely things that come with them.

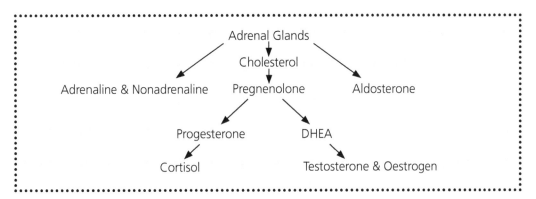

# How stress can affect fertility

Stress can directly affect fertility. (For that matter, stress can directly affect everything that sex hormones are required for. Ergo even if you couldn't care less about making babies, this is still relevant to you, so don't skip it!)

The main way stress affects your lady hormones is via CRF (see page 176). Studies have shown that enhanced CRF activity leads to a decrease in the production of gonadotropin releasing hormone (GnRH) from the hypothalamus. This has a flow-on effect of inhibiting the release of luteinising hormone (LH) from the pituitary, which is an essential hormone for ovulation in females.

In English: stress shuts down communication between your brain and your sex organs.

Numerous studies have shown that chronic stress can affect fertility by causing the following issues:

- Chronic anovulation (lack of ovulation).
- Hypothalamic amenorrhea/menstrual dysfunction.
- Pseudocyesis (phantom pregnancy, where you will have all of the signs of being pregnant, without actually being pregnant).
- Stress-related eating disorders.
- Hyperprolactinemia (high prolactin) and amenorrhea.
- Early pregnancy failure (studies have shown women with higher cortisol levels are more likely to experience early miscarriage).
- Oh, and it affects blokes too, so be sure to get your man sorted if you're trying to make a little human. It is 50:50, after all (well, at least in the beginning).

## OTHER BAD THINGS ABOUT STRESS

It's not just your sex hormones that are affected by stress. Check out this impressive list:

- Stress-induced cortisol release, on a regular basis, increases inflammation in the body. Hence stress can increase your risk of many chronic diseases, such as heart disease.
- Too much cortisol is also responsible for that belly fat you can't seem to budge, no matter how well you eat or drink.
- Chronic stress can disrupt your gut flora and, in turn, your overall health and wellbeing.
- Too much stress and cortisol can lead to adrenal fatigue and low energy.
- Stressing all the time can reduce your stomach acid and therefore your ability to properly break down and digest your food.
- Life really is too short to be sweating the small stuff all the time!

# IDENTIFYING ADRENAL FATIGUE

If you're really deep in the rabbit hole, you might be suffering from hypothalamic-pituitary-adrenal (HPA) dysfunction, which some folks refer to as adrenal fatigue, though this is often pooh-poohed by the medical community as not-a-real-condition.

A few signs that could point to you having adrenals in need of some TLC include:

- Feeling dizzy or faint when you go from lying down to standing up – bonus negative points if this happens when you go from sitting to standing.
- Sleep issues – trouble falling asleep, waking up multiple times throughout the night, struggling to drag your butt out of bed when the alarm goes off, feeling less-than-stellar despite getting a solid eight hours of sleep.
- Low blood sugar – think shaking, sweating, weakness, slight nausea, anxiousness, dizziness, blurred vision.
- You get hangry (hungry + angry) before a meal – or if you skip a meal; this could also appear as anxiety or irritability.
- You have a muffin top (belly fat) that wasn't there before – and won't shift despite your best diet and exercise attempts.
- You crave salty foods.
- Your memory is subpar – forget things much?
- You crash and burn at about 3 pm unless you have some sort of caffeinated or sugar-coated substance (and even that might not do the trick).
- Your recovery from exercise is poor and/or you are noticing your performance is decreasing – perhaps you're even noticing some niggles that weren't there before.
- You are getting sick more often.
- Sex drive? What sex drive?

# Tweaking your diet and lifestyle to relieve adrenal fatigue

If you have ticked several (hopefully not all) of the boxes for adrenal fatigue/ HPA dysregulation, you might want to really get serious about this whole stress management thing before you literally can't get out of bed. (I'm not joking, I have seen it happen.) We have discussed some of these strategies throughout the book, but here they are all in one place.

## Eat carbs – not too many, not too few

When you have adrenal fatigue, you need to support your body's blood sugar regulation. Too few carbs and your adrenals need to work to get blood sugar levels back up. Too many and blood sugar balance becomes difficult. Start with around 20 per cent (around 100 g in a 8368-kilojoule/2000-calorie diet) of your daily intake as carbs, as a minimum. You'll probably need more than this. Head back to the calorie and carb section in Chapter 5: Eat well to work out what this looks like in practical terms for you.

## Don't skimp on protein

Many women fail to include sufficient protein in their diet, regardless of whether or not their adrenals have copped a beating. Aim for at least 20 per cent (100 g in a 8368-kilojoule/2000-calorie diet) of your total intake. Having a decent chunk of protein with at least three of your meals should get you there.

You might find that starting the day with a higher protein brekkie will help keep your blood sugar levels stable over the day, and might even reduce your cravings. So, consider having steak for breakfast, maybe? With a bucketload of veggies to accompany it, please. If you're not into meat for breakfast you could have a couple of eggs, veggies and team these with a good quality protein shake. While you're at it, why not make it a green smoothie to sneak in a few more greens?

## Eat every three hours

The goal here is to avoid blood sugar-dips.

## Salt your meals

Unless you have high blood pressure, or you are eating a diet full of packaged and processed goo, it is okay to add some good quality sea salt to your meals. You will probably find it helps with your energy levels, too. Our bodies need salt. Too little is just as bad as too much.

## Ditch the stimulants

I know you really want (need?) that coffee to get you going, but over the long-term it's not going to do you any favours. Cut it out now, push through the few days of pain that accompany caffeine withdrawal and I promise you, you'll feel so much better in the long run, and your adrenals will thank you for it.

## Sleep

So important. Get at least seven to nine hours per night, in a dark room. If you need to take naps (and you can do so without getting fired), then do it. It won't be a forever thing, just while you are bringing your hormones back into balance.

## Exercise moderately

Favour the low-intensity activities such as walking, cycling, swimming, yoga, tai chi, dancing – preferably outside in the sunshine. I would strongly advise against HIIT in this situation. It's too stressful on your body.

### Consider supplementation

Ideally, work with a practitioner on this one. You shouldn't really take supplements willy-nilly. A few that can be helpful with tired adrenals include:

- Vitamin C.
- Ashwaganda (Indian ginsing).
- Rhodiola.
- Adrenal glandulars – yes, eating the adrenals of another animal. But before you go out and slaughter an animal, search for its kidneys and grab the little glands on top to add to your stew tonight. Also, know this: you can get these in capsule form. Hurrah!

# WORKING OUT YOUR SOURCES OF STRESS

If you are a stress addict, no matter how hard you try with squeaky-clean eating and smart training, you're probably not going to get the results you want, such as clear skin, abundant energy, optimal fertility, and effortless weight management – all of the lovely side effects that come with happy hormones. It's that simple. Stress affects *everything* in a negative way. I cannot express how important it is for you to incorporate daily stress management practices into your life. Please do not leave this one until last as it may in fact produce the fastest results for getting your hormones back on track. Manage the stress now, you won't regret it!

Are you stressed about being stressed now? Don't be. Just acknowledge it and be aware of your sources of stress, so you can then manage it more effectively.

Activity time! Where does your stress come from? How many of these can you tick off?

- Work
- Traffic
- Kids

- Partners
- Family (in-laws, anyone?)
- Money
- Illness/injury
- Other females
- Exercise (yes, exercise is a stressor – how much and what type you do determines whether it is a positive or negative stressor)
- Poor diet
- Can you list any others?

# FINDING WAYS TO RELIEVE STRESS

So you know that stress is no good, but how do you get it under control?

First of all, stop seeing stress as a good thing. Stop putting needless pressure on yourself to be, look and perform to perfection.

If you find yourself getting worked up, stop and think, 'Will this matter in five years from now?' If the answer is 'no', then calm down, my friend.

Stress management doesn't mean you have to sit cross-legged in lotus position for an hour by a fish pond with colourful koi every day. That's just not realistic for many (or most) people. If truth be told, I have been trying to establish a regular meditation practice for five years and still only make it to the middle of January with this New Year's resolution. I'm definitely not saying you shouldn't meditate. If you can, then more power to you.

There are loads of practices you can implement on a daily basis to reduce stress. It all comes down to personal preference, really. Check out the myriad ways on the next page that you can reduce your stress levels and get yourself into a state of zen (or at least a little less frazzled and more capable of managing your response to stressors).

# Sex

Yes, you should be having sex; especially when having lady-hormone issues. It's fun and reduces stress. If you're single, you can still experience the stress-reducing benefits of orgasm, which is beyond the scope of this book.

# Laughter

It really is the best medicine. Have a good chuckle with your nearest and dearest, or maybe just sit down and watch some *Family Guy*. And remember, as Norman Cousins says, 'Hearty laughter ... is a good way to jog internally without having to go outdoors.'

# Play

Speaking of laughter, you are never too old to get a little silly! Go and visit a kid's playground and jump on the swings, climbing equipment and flying fox. If it's raining, go and jump in the puddles. If it's autumn, go and kick the leaves around. If it sounds silly and childish, go and do it with gay abandon!

# Yoga

Probably not bikram, though. Choose something like yin, hatha or vinyasa. Again, branch out and go for a style that soothes your soul.

# Meditation

You might find it helpful to get started with an app such as HeadSpace. And remember, don't let the perfect get in the way of the good. Rather than put the pressure on yourself to start with an hour of deep meditation in an ashram in India, why not just start with a few minutes at home, either seated or lying down. You can't go wrong, so just go with the flow.

Many people tend to get hung up with not being able to clear their mind 100 per cent of thoughts when they try meditating. That's okay, it's not about being completely zenned out to start with. Simply notice your thoughts, try not to hold on to them, and experiment with following the movement of your breath as much as possible. As much as you might think you do, you can't suck at meditation. There is no prize for being the best at this, yet the personal rewards you reap from simply sitting and doing nothing but breathing for a moment or two are endless.

## Breathe, baby

This is one of the easiest and fastest ways to activate your parasympathetic (rest, digest and reproduce) nervous system. The best time to start with deep belly breathing is first thing in the morning, before you even get out of bed. As soon as you wake up, place your hands on your belly and feel it rise and fall with each breath. Close your eyes if it helps, but try not to drift back to sleep. And don't blame me if you end up late for work!

Try for ten deep breaths. It should only take a few minutes, so no excuses please. That's it! Day started on the right foot. This is also a good one for when you're stuck in traffic, when your annoying co-worker is giving you the heebie-jeebies, or when you find yourself getting a little worked up in any other potentially stressful situation.

## Make gratitude your only attitude

It is hard (or even impossible) to be negative or stressed out when you are practising gratitude. My dear (smart) hubby suggested to me a while ago that I should start a gratitude journal where I write three things down each night that I am grateful for.

I can honestly say that practising gratitude has had a *huge* impact on my life, and that of my clients. Personally, I notice that I feel more optimistic and that more positivity is drawn into my life. I appreciate all of the little things that I have, such as clean water, sunshine, and a well-functioning, fertile body that allows me to live a full and wholesome life. I feel truly lucky to live the life that I do. Do you?

Let's take a detour with a little story, shall we?

I remember a couple of years ago having a moment of negativity about the cellulite on my thighs. Then I watched a documentary about a photographer who had both of his legs blown off by a mine in Afghanistan. Did he sit at home and wallow? Not at all, he got back out there and carried on with his life. It made me realise that I should be grateful that I *have* legs. Who really cares if they have a few dimples on them?! This really is a first-world problem! Sometimes we need to put things into a bit of perspective, don't you think?

So, each night, write down three things that you are grateful for. Don't get too caught up in it. They don't have to be grand. Some things you might be grateful for include:

- The sun shining – or the rain!
- Your warm bed.
- Your toothbrush.
- The support of your friends and family.
- The ability to access fresh, wholesome food and water (a luxury that many cannot afford, yet we so easily take for granted).
- The opportunity to spend time outside.
- Having a productive day at work.

## Affirmations

This might sound a bit crunchy-hippy to you and, admittedly, if you'd have suggested it to me five years ago I probably would have thought so too. However, having put it into practice over the years, both personally and professionally, I can tell you it is well worth it. For most people, affirmations work an absolute treat! The effort is minimal, and you don't even have to say them out loud if you're worried about looking like a loon. Simply repeat them in your head, or write them out, or both for extra brownie points!

Affirmations are positive declarations that describe a desired situation, which are often repeated until they get impressed on the subconscious mind. This process pushes the subconscious mind to take action and try to make the positive statement come true.

So often we will repeat negative statements in our mind, which only further cultivates negativity, poor self-esteem and frustration. How often do you find yourself saying things like:

- 'I'm fat and ugly.'
- 'Why should anyone love me?'
- 'My body is broken.'
- 'There is never enough time in the day.'
- 'I'm soooo stressed.'
- 'I really hate my [insert body part here].'
- 'Life is too hard.'
- 'Nothing ever goes my way.'
- 'I'll never be able to afford [X].'

Sadly, I hear these sorts of negative proclamations all the time, and they aren't doing us any favours. Negative chatter (either out loud or in your mind) will never lead to positive outcomes. How can you expect to be happy when you always have a negative mindset and are focusing on how terrible everything is? Let's turn that frown upside down, okay? A few of my favourite affirmations include:

- 'I am strong, healthy and fertile.'
- 'I easily fall pregnant with a strong and healthy child' (– if that's what you're aiming for).
- 'I love my body.'
- 'I am beautiful and worthy of love.'

- ❧ 'There is plenty of time in the day to get everything done.'
- ❧ 'My body is functional' – this is a great one for focusing on all of the wonderful things your body can do, as opposed to how your body looks or how you perceive it to look. Chances are you think things are worse than they actually are.
- ❧ 'I have a wonderful life.'
- ❧ 'Everything in my life is exactly as it should be at this moment.'
- ❧ 'I have a great relationship with money.'
- ❧ 'Abundance is drawn to me from all angles' (– this and the previous one are great for those of you who draw most of your stress from financial worries).

You can make up whatever you want. Just think about how you want things to be in the present tense and create a statement to reflect this. Then repeat, repeat, repeat!

At first you might not believe these declarations, but stick with it. Eventually you will notice the mental shift followed finally by a physical shift.

## Spend time with animals and/or children

Preferably when they're not going mental ... Get down on the floor and roll around with them. Hug them. Kiss them. Laugh with them. Everyone's a winner in this scenario!

## Immerse yourself in nature

Go for a hike! Swim at the beach! Do some gardening! Why am I yelling these statements? Because it is important. We spend too much time indoors and not enough time outside getting our daily dose of vitamin N (nature). I am aware that it's not actually a vitamin, but should be in the sense that it is vital for life. Spending time in nature can be incredibly healing – mentally, emotionally, physically and spiritually.

## Socialise with friends

In real life. Not through Facebook. Not through email. Not through text. These don't count. Make a date, stick to it (don't be flakey), and enjoy some invaluable face-to-face time with your besties.

## Call someone

When was the last time you picked up the phone and just had a good natter about anything and everything? This can be great for getting your mind off those things that are causing you stress. Plus it'll be beneficial for the relationship. Chances are your buddy on the other end of the line could do with a good chat, too, and will appreciate you taking the initiative to call. Go on!

## Hug it out for health and happiness

One of the easiest ways to improve your health and happiness is simply by giving someone a hug. How so?

A psychotherapist named Virginia Satir once said 'We need four hugs a day for survival. We need eight hugs a day for maintenance. We need twelve hugs a day for growth.' (Maybe stick this on your fridge as a friendly reminder)

Twelve hugs! That's a lot of hugs! You might actually have to head out into a busy mall offering free hugs to get to this level. Or you could walk around and wrap your arms around everyone in your office. Or a stranger. They might think you're weird (isn't that sad?), but I bet it also makes them smile.

So why are hugs so good? They stimulate the release of oxytocin – your bliss hormone. This chemical is made in your hypothalamus and released from your pituitary gland. Oxytocin has been shown to reduce your blood pressure and heart rate (thereby improving your heart health). It can lower cortisol levels (this is what we want and need to feel all yummy and sexy), can ease depression, boost immunity and help fight fatigue. Wowsers! All of this with a little hugging action!

And this: full body hugs (not entirely sure what this means – legs wrapped around too?) can decrease feelings of loneliness and fear, improve self-esteem, reduce tension and boost your mood.

For extra benefits, make it a long, extended, slightly awkward hug. (Don't you hate it when you mess up the finish time? Either you hold on too long or pull away too soon ...) If you're not up for the long holds, that's okay. A quick hug is better than no hug.

## Take a bath

Take in a good book or trashy mag (leave work outside the bathroom, please), maybe a cup of chamomile tea, and soak away your stressors until your fingers and toes go wrinkly like a prune.

For extra calming benefits, and a little detoxification boost, add in a cup of Epsom salts. This is also a wonderful way to get some magnesium into your system, which is a mineral most of us are deficient in, yet it is essential for over 300 processes in the body!

If you really want to set the mood, don't hesitate to dim the lights, fire up some candles and possibly even pop on some relaxing music. Ahhhh, bliss!

## Have a cuppa

Yep, put the kettle on, kick off your heels and get ready to have a chill-out moment with a soothing cup of tea. Studies have shown that enjoying a cup of tea can reduce stress and anxiety not just by drinking the good stuff, but also through the ritual of preparing it.

Most research has shown these benefits to be reaped from your average cup of English Breakfast (which those crazy Kiwis call Gumboot Tea here in NZ). However, I would suggest steering clear of the caffeine if you're already a bit frazzled, and opt for a yummy herbal tea.

A few tasty (and some not-so-tasty, but still beneficial) tea treats that are helpful for tired adrenals include:

- Licorice tea (my favourite)
- Chamomile tea
- Ashwaganda (Indian ginseng)
- Tulsi tea (aka holy basil)
- Valerian (though it could make you sleepy, so don't drive under the influence)
- Lemon balm
- Passion flower
- Hops (and no, beer is not a good substitute for the tea)
- Kava kava.

Or, you could just visit your local health food store, or even the supermarket, and grab yourself a sleepytime tea – many companies have cottoned on to these blends.

# Sing

In the shower. In the car. In the forest. By yourself. With others. To others. The louder and crazier the better! (I like to sing along to the **Pitch Perfect** soundtrack. Don't judge me.)

# Dance

Like no-one is watching ...

# Get a massage

Or other spa treatment. I was chatting with a lady the other day, aged 33, who had never had a massage/facial/pedi. Now that is just insane! Schedule some time (and money), and head to your local spa or beauty salon and treat yo'self!

## Read a good book

Or a magazine. Just kick back for a bit, and be okay if you fall asleep mid-reading – chances are you need a little kip.

## Go to the movies

Get your girlfriends together for a movie night, or don't be afraid to head there by yourself.

## Grab yourself some Derwents and get arty

Adult colouring-in books! Have you tried them? It's what all the cool kids are doing these days. They are a great way to zone out for a bit and head into a kind of meditative state (without actually meditating).

## Smile

Here's a challenge for you ... Smile at two people that you walk past during your day. Complete strangers. Hopefully they'll smile back. (If not, chase them down and ask what their problem is. Kidding! Don't do that.) Maybe even say good morning. It'll give you (and them) a warm fuzzy feeling to kickstart your day, and theirs.

## Have a social media detox

Smart science-peeps have reported that the more time you spend on Facebook or other social media, the more likely you are to experience depressive symptoms. At the very least, you will most likely experience a bit of FOMO (fear of missing out), which isn't going to make you feel great about your life. So, switch off for a few days. The world is not going to end, and chances are not much will change in the online world in your absence.

I would recommend having a few days off social media at least every few months. If this scares you, then at least don't touch your phone until you head out the door in the morning, after you have had a nice, peaceful breakfast.

## Be okay with saying no

Try not to fall into the trap of saying 'yes' to every request, every offer, every demand. Otherwise you will surely find yourself snowed under with a mammoth to-do list and stress levels to boot! It's okay to say no sometimes. It might feel weird at first, and maybe take a bit of practice, but over time you will learn to prioritise your own health first, which will in turn improve your relationships with others.

## Avoid people who stress you out

I'm sure you can think of at least a couple of people who irk you. Perhaps it is your mother-in-law, or a co-worker, or a friend of a friend. Whoever it is, if you find yourself feeling crappy after spending time with them, then tell them to take a hike. Kidding. Seriously though be kind and considerate but keep your interactions with them to a minimum. Some might be harder than others. If it is impossible to avoid them, come back to your happy place and just focus on breathing. And remember, as William Gibson says:

*Before you diagnose yourself with depression or low self-esteem, first make sure that you are not, in fact, just surrounding yourself with assholes.*

# Say goodbye to female competition

I think female competition is one of those things that boggles the minds of men. And so it should; it is ridiculous. The ancestral woman would not compete with other females for who had the best body, the best outfit, the best hair do or the best job. The ancestral woman spent time with, and supported, other women. Social and emotional support is hugely important in helping to reduce stress levels. And let's be honest, there is nothing sexy about bitchiness, right?

# Sleep

Ahh, blissful sleep. Unfortunately, as I write this, my darling daughter is teething, and so sleep eludes me. And don't I know it!

A lack of sleep is not only stressful on your body, it can mess with your health, big time – and that means your hormones! I could write a whole book on sleep, but instead I'll just offer a few tips to help you get the best quality sleep possible:

1  Do not use electronics one to two hours prior to bed time. I'm talking smartphones, iPads and e-readers, computers and TV. The blue light emitted from these triggers the release of cortisol and blocks the release of melatonin (your sleep hormone).
2  If you must use electronics, grab yourself some blue-blocker/amber-tinted glasses to wear at night.
3  Sleep in a slightly cool environment. Not a sauna. Not an ice-house.
4  Try not to go to bed on a full stomach. Leave a couple of hours post-dinner.
5  Avoid sugar and caffeine at night, as these can be too stimulating.
6  Have carbs with dinner (gasp!) – carbs can help with the production of tryptophan, which eventually converts to melatonin.
7  When you wake up in the morning, head outside into the sunshine without your sunnies on to help regulate your sleep–wake cycles.
8  Minimise alcohol consumption, as this can make your sleep junky.

**9** Take magnesium before bed.

**10** Avoid intense exercise in the evening. Instead, opt for gentle, restorative activity.

**11** Try to go to bed and wake up at the same time every day.

I'm sure there are more ways to stop being a stress-head. Just think about what you find fun and enjoyable, and chances are they will also be great stress relievers!

When should you do your stress-relieving activities? All the time, ideally. However, the best time to start is in the morning. Just do something small to reduce your stress and energise your day.

As a final note on stress management, if you take nothing else from this chapter: *embrace imperfection*. Not everything in your life has to be perfect. Just let it go.

## Recap time

- ❧ **Stress is not your friend and can undo all of the hormone-balancing work you have done with diet and exercise.**
- ❧ **Chronic stress depletes sex hormones, negatively affects fertility (in women and men) and can increase your risk of chronic disease.**
- ❧ **If you have adrenal fatigue (from excess and/or extended stress), you will need to be diligent with stress management every day, along with making specific dietary and exercise tweaks to your life, to avoid falling in a burnt-out heap.**
- ❧ **Daily stress management can work wonders for happifying your hormones.Check back to the myriad suggestions in this chapter, there's something for everyone!**

Now that you're all cool, calm and collected, I think this is a great time to talk about a bit of self-lovin'. My favourite (and possibly the most important) chapter is up next.

# BE KIND

*For some reason, we are truly convinced that if we criticise ourselves,*
*the criticism will lead to change. If we are harsh, we believe we will end*
*up being kind. If we shame ourselves, we believe we end up loving*
*ourselves. It has never been true, not for a moment,*
*that shame leads to love. Only love leads to love.*
– Geneen Roth

This chapter is so important, yet I bet that most of you aren't getting into the whole self-love thing. Or perhaps you are, but not really regularly enough. Or maybe you are doing it all day, every day. Well done, you.

If you don't love, respect and appreciate yourself (body, mind and spirit), then your chances of nourishing yourself appropriately for hormonal balance, through eating well, training smart and managing stress, are diminished. We'll chat more about this shortly.

On top of this, when you focus on your apparent flaws, this leads to a negative mindset, which can be a very stressful state to hang out in. And, as you know (because we just went through it), stress is the Grinch of happy hormones.

In this chapter, you'll learn all about what self-love actually is, we'll dive deeper into why it is important for happiness (not just happy hormones, but real, whole-body happiness right down to your core), and of course, you'll find an abundance of ways to practise self-love and compassion.

# WHAT IS SELF-LOVE?

Well, it's pretty self-explanatory, really. Self-love is all about showing *yourself* some love. The kind of love that you would show a cherished family member, a child, or a best friend. The kind of love that might make you feel a bit weird at first. But it shouldn't. It will only feel odd as we are so out of practice. Self-love is often caught up with perceived notions of narcissism – that you are self-centred or full of yourself. Please let go of these negative connotations now. Just because you are showing kindness, understanding, and non-judgement towards yourself, does not mean that you will simultaneously be showing complete disregard and lack of empathy for others. Here's a little secret: your heart is big enough to love yourself and others!

Self-love is not something that can be bought. Nor is it something that can be handed to you on a silver platter. And it's not something that will come out of a new relationship. Or new clothes. Or (definitely not) a number on a scale that you might think of as desirable.

Self-love is something that is acquired, and something that grows over time, as a result of you taking action *all the time*. Though this might seem like hard work, it really isn't, and the benefits you will reap will far outweigh any potential costs.

Self-love is about valuing your own happiness and wellbeing. It is about meeting your own emotional needs on a continuous basis.

These are all round-about definitions. I can't really express exactly what self-love is, as it will be different for each and every one of you. By this, I mean that you will all have your own unique ways of showing yourself a little lovin'. There is no wrong way to show yourself love and compassion. If it makes you feel all warm and fuzzy, then chances are you're on the money, and should keep doing what you're doing.

# WHY SELF-LOVE AND COMPASSION?

If you don't love and respect yourself, if you refuse to be compassionate with and kind to yourself, chances are you're not likely to look after yourself in other ways, such as with diet, exercise and stress management. Once you acknowledge your worthiness – yes, you *are* worthy – then I can guarantee you will be more inclined to look after yourself, and your hormones, in a holistic, and sustainable way each and every day. Not only this, but you'll be happier and more confident in your own skin. You will have a much better body image (and I am sure most of us can benefit from this). You won't always be trying to fix yourself by losing more and more weight, or getting rid of the last little dimple on your upper thigh, or covering up your perceived flaws with caked-on make-up.

A few other benefits of practising self-love and compassion include:

- Improved self-esteem.
- Greater life satisfaction.
- Increased happiness.
- Greater resilience and improved ability to deal with difficult situations (such as divorce or job loss)
- Decreased risk of developing mental illnesses such as depression and anxiety.
- Boosted optimism.
- Better relationships (– you know the saying, you can't expect to love anyone else until you can love yourself).

Sounds good, doesn't it? But perhaps it seems unachievable? It is unachievable if you don't put some steps in place to try to achieve it.

*And if I asked you to name all the things that you love,*
*how long would it take for you to name yourself?*
– @wellandgoodnyc

Now I know this is going to be a sticking point for many of you. It was for me too. I hope the suggestions in this chapter will help, but know that it is probably not going to be a straight and narrow road. There may be days when you feel frumpy or negative about yourself. And that's okay. This is where the compassion part comes in. The key is to persevere, and slowly those negative days will be drowned out by the positive. Be gentle with yourself and, again, it's not about striving for perfection.

Fun side note: practising self-love and compassion will help with perfectionism. When things don't go exactly as you would like them to, you'll be okay with it, and less likely to beat yourself, or anyone else, up.

# SUGGESTIONS FOR PRACTISING SELF-LOVE AND COMPASSION

Don't feel you need to do all of these (though please be my guest if you want to). Simply pick one or two practices that resonate with you. Start with these few for a little while, and then when you are comfortable with them, and start to notice how amazing they make you feel, why not toss in another practice? Layer it up! The more the merrier – literally.

## Change how you think, and talk, about food

So often I hear foods referred to as either good or bad. Food should not have morality, as when it does, we imprint this morality on ourselves when we eat such foods. When we eat bad foods, we then feel guilty and say we have been bad. This is not helpful. It's just another way to make us feel bad about ourselves, increase stress levels, and feel like we are failing and need to do better.

Instead, think about how food feels for you. Food is fuel – think about foods that will give you energy, foods that will nourish you from the inside-out, foods that help balance your hormones. And on those occasions when you have some not-so-healthy foods, be okay with it. Don't feel you need to hide away and be ashamed of it. Eat it slowly and mindfully. (Remember reading about this in Chapter 5: Eat Well?) Enjoy it. Then move on. There is no point in beating yourself up about it; it's not going to change the fact that you ate it. Nor is that one experience going to make a significant contribution, as we often expect it will, to your weight or your health in general. That's right, you will not gain weight or develop diabetes from the odd piece of cake! It's more about what you eat every day, as opposed to what you eat every now and then. So you can have your cake and eat it too!

## Do not compare yourself to others

Comparison is the thief of joy, haven't you heard? (Thanks, Teddy Roosevelt.) When you compare yourself to others, or judge others, you are essentially judging yourself. There are no winners here. Often, we compare ourselves with others whom we perceive to have something better than us, which only serves to make us feel worse about ourselves.

Instead, celebrate who you are. You are uniquely awesome. No-one has the exact same qualities as you, and that is a good thing! Because if we were all the same, how boring would that be?

Embrace your own personal journey. That's all that matters, really, and also the only one in which you truly know what is going on.

On that note, try not to compare yourself to your former self either. This is especially important for anyone recovering from conditions such as hypothalamic amenorrhea or eating disorders. Possibly adrenal fatigue, too. Remember, to recover from these situations, you will most likely need to decrease your exercise, eat more, and possibly put on weight and/or body fat. Constantly referring to how you used to look will only put the brakes on your willingness to move forward with healing. Put things into perspective: yes, you may have been able to see your abs, but were you healthy? Were you even happy? Personally, when I had abs and was a lean, mean, fighting machine, I was not healthy (infertile, brittle bones, low energy, no sex drive), nor was I happy!

> *You know when you stare at a word for so long it starts to not look like a word anymore, like something is wrong with it? I think this is the same thing girls do to their bodies.*
> – Frankly Cats on Tumblr

## Re-evaluate who you follow on social media

Put down this book right now and have a look through your image-based social media (such as Instagram, Pinterest and Facebook). When you come across a picture that makes you feel bad about yourself – perhaps it makes you feel as though you should be leaner/prettier/exercising more/eating less – hit the 'unfollow' button. I'm talking about a lot of the 'thinspo', 'fitspo' and 'strongisthenewskinny' sort of accounts.

Instead, start to follow people who make you feel inspired, joyful and make you yell, 'Hell yeah! I am freakin' awesome!'

> *Perhaps we should love ourselves so fiercely that when others see us, they know exactly how it should be done.*
> – Rudy Francisco

## Throw out the scales

When you weigh yourself, all you're really weighing is your self-esteem. Here's what the scales can't tell you and why you should say goodbye right now:

- ❦ How healthy you are.
- ❦ How happy you are.

- ❧ How nourished you are.
- ❧ What your body is physically capable of.
- ❧ Your energy level/vitality.
- ❧ Your worth as a person.

Think about your last encounter with the scales. I bet before weighing-in you were checking yourself out in the mirror thinking, 'Oh yeah, I look hot today! I'm definitely going to weigh X kg (with 'X' referring to your desired weight, or less).' You're quite chuffed with yourself at this point. You feel sexy. You feel confident. It's a good day.

Then you step on that nasty little box of hate and the number that flashes back at you is higher than you expected. Day ruined. You look back in the mirror and think, 'I'm so fat/ugly/unworthy.' Self-esteem squashed. You proceed to get changed into one of your fat-day outfits and slump out the door with sad face in place.

How on earth does that happen? How do we even rationalise going from one extreme to the other in a matter of minutes, all thanks to a stupid little box on the ground? The answer is we don't – our crazy female brain takes over and all rationality goes out the window. So the solution? Don't put yourself through the senseless punishment!

Some better ways to measure your progress include:

- ❧ Go by how you feel, not how you look (shock horror).
- ❧ Reflect on changes in your performance – can you lift more weight? Run further? Dance for longer without running out of breath? Stand on your head in yoga? These are all worthy of recognition. Much more worthy than your weight, in my opinion!
- ❧ Take photos of yourself (but not if recovering from HA or eating disorders) – weekly, monthy, bi-monthly – you choose. This way you will have a bit more of an objective view of how you look. The problem with the scales is that they do not differentiate between muscle and fat, nor do they account for the fluid that we ladies can sometimes hold on to. So you might be putting on muscle and losing fat, but the scales don't shift in

the direction you expect them to. The difference with using pictures throughout your journey is that you will be able to see, loud and clear, this increased muscle mass and changed body composition. You don't have to get professional photos, nor do you have to show anyone if you don't want to. Just use your smartphone and take some selfies in the bathroom.

❧ How do your clothes fit? This will also provide more of an accurate reflection than the scales. Although, do be aware that if you are doing quite a bit of weight training, your muscles will increase (though probably not to Madonna-arms level, so don't freak out), and some of your clothes might be a bit tighter.

Also realise that your goals might take a little while to achieve. So let go of perfectionism and instant gratification – good things take time. Think about how long it took you to get into the situation you are currently in that you would like to change. Chances are it will take just as long, possibly even longer, to get yourself out of it and into the place you want to be: (That's if you're doing it in a healthy, sustainable manner). This is where that whole self-compassion and understanding comes into play.

# Develop self-respect

Speak to yourself as if you were speaking to a best friend. Would you tell your best friend 'you're fat', 'you're ugly', 'you're not worthy'? No? You probably wouldn't even say those words to a stranger, right? Then why say them to yourself? Your body has done more for you than anyone else will ever do. Show a little respect.

# Use your affirmations

Head back to Chapter 7: Manage stress where I spoke about affirmations. Also, if you want to get more into this practice, I can highly recommend checking out the work of both Louise Hay and Gabrielle Bernstein.

# Have a self-love ritual

Have a practice that you can do when you're really in a funk. This will be your happy place to help get your mojo back. Something you might like is a bit of a self-pampering session. Grab the candles, run a bath, have a soak and a cup of tea. When you get out, why not give yourself a loving massage with some beautiful oils. Think of it as a thanks, from you to your body, for all that it does for you. It's the only one you have, so treat it well.

Something else that I find to be a nice practice, especially when you're having a negative body image day, is to do a little thing that I like to call 'The Body Love Scan'. Here's how it goes: while you're still in the nuddy (aka naked), stand in front of the mirror and, working from top to toe, place your hands over each body part and say, 'I love my [insert body part here].' So you will start with your hair, hands on head and say, 'I love my hair.' And yes, this will also involve saying, 'I love my boobs', 'I love my tummy' and 'I love my thighs'. Spend a little extra time on those parts you've been most negative about over the years.

# Work with your body, not against it

Try meeting your body where it is at, right now, rather than where you, or society, think it should be. Let go of any unrealistic expectations. Listen to your body and respond with love and kindness. Stop trying to beat your body into submission in order to achieve a physique that you are not meant to have.

I have personally realised that I will never have a thigh gap. And I'm okay with that. (Really, thigh gaps are mostly for thirteen-year-old prepubescent girls, or boys for that matter! So just let it go.)

Forcing your body to do anything will only create greater resistance. Start to develop flow and everything will eventually fall into place.

*You look how you look. Be comfortable. What are you going to do? Be hungry every single day to make other people happy? That's just dumb.*
– Jennifer Lawrence

## Move your body on a daily basis

Moving your body on a regular basis (and no, I don't mean exercise for the sake of burning kilojoules or getting stronger, I mean movement for movement's sake), is a great way to nourish every cell in your body. Why not just start with a little stretching as a way to say 'thank you' to your body? I like to do this at night-time; it's a nice way to wind down for the day.

Also revisit the Chapter 6: Train Smart to nab some other ideas about movement.

## Create a 'What's good about me' list

Think of all the things, unrelated to your appearance, that are wonderful about you. Are you kind? Write it down! Are you funny? Write it down! Are you creative? Write it down! You get the picture. If you're struggling to think of anything, don't beat yourself up. Just go and have a chat with a loved one and ask them to tell you what's good about you.

Once you have your list, write each point out on separate post-it notes and stick them up around your house as a friendly reminder of just how awesome you are! Don't skip this part – your positive attributes should be pointed out to you all the time until you walk past each note and say, 'Yeah! I *am* awesome!'

Also, try this: whenever someone gives you a compliment, write it down. Straight away so you don't forget about it! Then add that to your note collection. And if someone says something not-so-nice to you, get into the practice of just letting it go. It is more a reflection of their own insecurities than anything about you. So forgive them, as holding a grudge is like drinking poison yourself and expecting the other person to die. Only you will suffer, as they carry on with their life, completely oblivious to the fact.

## Have a spring clean of your clothes

Do you really need an excuse to go shopping? Throw out all of your clothes that don't make you feel 100 per cent remarkable, and replace them with some nice, shiny new ones. Out with the old, in with the new – clothes and thoughts!

## Do something you are good at

Participating in something that you are good at is a sure-fire way to boost your self-esteem, and bring out the best version of you.

## Just let it go

I have said it before, and I'll say it again. Be okay with imperfection. Perfectionism serves no-one and can be absolutely stifling. It's also a great way to dampen your day if everything is not going exactly how it should be.

There really is no such thing as perfect – when you get to that point where you thought everything would be perfect, I bet you will find something else to pick out that needs changing.

*Imperfection is beauty, madness is genius and it's better to be absolutely ridiculous than absolutely boring.*
– Marilyn Monroe

# Pay attention to your thoughts

Are you constantly telling yourself negative, derogatory things? Do you walk around thinking 'I'm so fat', 'I'm so ugly'? For a day, each time you think, or say, something negative about yourself, write it down. At the end of the day, reflect on your list of mean-girl comments. Hopefully your list isn't too long (ideally it should be non-existent). But if it is quite extensive, how does it make you feel? I suspect a bit of reality might bubble to the surface about how nasty, and unproductive, your words have been.

Have a think about how you can be kinder to yourself the following day. Over time, try to drown out the nasty with the nice. Repeat after me: 'I am fabulous! I am beautiful. I am worthy. I am loved.' The more you say these sorts of statements, the more you will feel them.

Why not try running through these mantras as soon as you wake up – while you're doing your deep belly breathing! At the end of the day, thank your fine self for being so damn magnificent.

I love this quote from Danielle LaPorte on self-criticism. Read it. Memorise it. Be inspired by it to make change:

*'Self-criticism is not "love", and it is certainly not indifferent. It's a form of hatred. And when I name that, when I see it for what it is (raw and uncomfortable and saddening ...) when I refuse to sugar-coat self-criticism, judgement, agitation, and constantly trying to improve myself, then I'm one quantum leap closer to freedom. Out of the swamp. Grounded in love.'*

Hopefully that tugs a little at your heartstrings and gives you the nudge you need to speak with words of warmth to yourself.

Forgive yourself on days that have not gone so swimmingly, and perhaps you weren't quite as friendly to yourself as you could have been. Tomorrow is another day and another opportunity to practise kindness.

# Focus on the positives

If you find yourself stuck in a funk about, for example, the shape of your body changing as you recover from whipping it into a state that it was not designed to be in, try writing out a list of pros and cons.

After about three months of making changes to recover from HA, which required me to put on weight (especially body fat) and say goodbye to my washboard stomach, I decided to write such a list, which looked something like this.

Cons:

- My jeans don't fit me anymore. (Actually, it was only one pair that didn't fit – the rest were pretty good with their stretchability. Yes, it's a word.)
- I probably won't be called up by Victoria to replace Miranda as her new Angel.

Pros:

- I have boobs. This might seem insignificant to all you well-endowed ladies out there, but coming from someone who has always struggled to fill an A-cup (don't laugh) it's pretty exciting.
- I am so much more in tune with my body now. I listen to how it feels and I respond with understanding and respect.
- My nails are thick and strong.
- My grey hairs have disappeared, seriously! I didn't think it possible, but my hairdresser will quite happily tell you I used to have quite a few greys!
- My skin and eyes are clearer than they have ever been. And I don't use fancy skincare products. I use olive oil and soap. Maybe a little rosehip oil in the winter. That's it!
- I feel stronger. I can lift heavier weights in the gym, despite doing less exercise overall.
- I have unbelievable energy. Eating more = more nutrients pulsing through my body.
- I feel more comfortable in my body. Seriously. For the first time in about fifteen years, I feel good. Really good.

- ❧ My hubby still finds me sexy.
- ❧ My friends still want to hang out with me.
- ❧ I am now in the position to help others and be a positive role model for them, which was my intention for this book.

So it would seem that this whole change business ain't so bad after all. Admittedly, there were days when I would feel a bit shabby and want to go back to my svelte ways. But slowly, the good days crowded out the bad. These things take time. And they can be scary. Which is why you should not feel as though you have to do it alone. Get support; tell your friends and family. It's okay not to be perfect; people will probably love you more for your imperfections! And above all, hold your own hand along the way. Be gentle with yourself and reflect on the positives – they are always there – you just need to look.

## Express yourself

We all have feelings. That's what makes us human! Sometimes, though, we have a tendency to shove any yucky feelings under the carpet, and pretend they aren't there. When we do this, these feelings fester and create mould under the carpet, causing greater problems in the long run. What should you do instead? Express your emotions! If you're feeling angry, that's okay – let it out! Preferably choose a manner that won't hurt another person, either emotionally or physically. You might like to take up boxing as a way to release any feelings of anger or aggression. Or you could try journalling if that tickles your fancy.

If you're sad, cry. There is nothing worse than holding in a good cry. If you don't want to do it in front of anyone, go and find a quiet spot and just let it out. No holding back.

# Fill in this picture

And stick it on your wall.

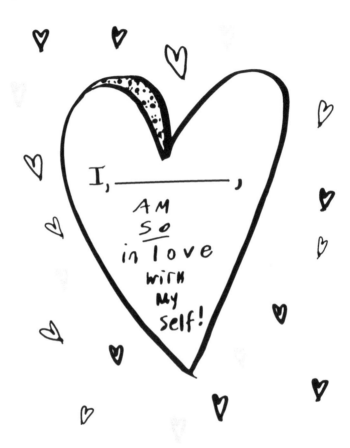

I, _____, AM SO in love wiTH My self!

## Give yourself permission to play

As adults, we are way too serious. When was the last time you played? And I mean really let your hair down and got stupid-silly? The kind of silly that an uptight person would scoff at (but secretly they wish they could join in)?

Go on! Find your inner child and go crazy.

# Eat dark chocolate

Because why not? In case you need some convincing (doubtful), here are a few fun facts that you might not have known about why dark chocolate (cacao) makes you feel so loved up:

- Raw cacao is rich in phenethylamin (PEA), which is a feel-good neurotransmitter (brain messenger) that is responsible for the feeling of love!
- Cacao also contains tryptophan, an amino acid that serves as a precursor for serotonin, our happy hormone, which is often depleted in people who suffer from depression.
- Cacao is the only food source of anandamide, aka the Bliss Chemical, a neurotransmitter responsible for the feeling of bliss. Some research is suggesting that this chemical may be useful for treating anxiety and depression

Know this: milk chocolate (or white chocolate) is not chocolate. It is chocolate-flavoured sugar. Go dark all the way – ideally 85 per cent or higher. Or why not make your own from cacao powder? Check out the recipes for Raw Sesame Fudge (page 240) or Chocolate Avocado Mousse (page 242).

# Get more sleep

There's a reason sleep deprivation is used as a form of torture. Don't do it to yourself.

# Don't be afraid to seek help

Looking after yourself, loving yourself and being kind to yourself can be super-difficult if you have been doing the opposite for an extended period of time. Don't be swayed by the challenge and put it in the too-hard basket. If you're struggling to get on board with this crunchy hippy stuff by yourself, it is completely reasonable to seek out professional help in the form of a psychologist or counsellor. There is no shame in that. You deserve to be happy, to be loved, to feel accepted and secure, to exude confidence. Invest in yourself for a healthier and happier future.

What do you think? Ready to start loving yourself more and reaping the benefits? Exciting, isn't it? So start right away. Not tomorrow. Not Monday. Right now. Go!

*Live with intention. Walk to the edge. Listen hard. Practise wellness. Play with abandon. Laugh. Choose with no regret. Continue to learn. Appreciate your friends. Do what you love. Live as if this is all there is.*
– Mary Anne Radmacher

## Recap time

- ❧ Self-love and compassion are essential to develop self-worth and self-respect, which will put you in the best position to nourish yourself, and your hormones, with good food, movement and stress management.
- ❧ Self-love is not about narcissism. When you love yourself, you are also better able to love others – your heart has an infinite capacity for love.
- ❧ With self-love and compassion come loads of benefits, including boosted self-esteem, better body image, better relationships, reduced stress and increased happiness.
- ❧ There are so many ways to practise self-love and compassion, including letting go of comparisons, getting in touch with your inner child through play, and eating dark chocolate.
- ❧ Love is the thing!

# RECIPES

*People who love to eat are always the best people.*
– Julia Child

## BREAKFAST

When it comes to hormone balance, I do like to recommend people eat a decent breakfast. I'm not of the opinion that breakfast is the most important meal of the day, but I am of the opinion that breakfast is the most important meal of the day to not mess up. It can make or break your whole day.

If you start your day with cereal and low-fat yoghurt, a skinny flat white, and some toast with margarine and vegemite, you can expect your blood sugar levels to go all over the place right from the word go. You have learned in this book how crazy blood sugars can mess with your adrenals (important for those of you with adrenal fatigue, infertility and hypothalamic amenorrhea), and how they create drama with insulin (I'm looking at you, PCOS, weight loss resistance and diabetes), so it's wise to start your day with a nourishing meal.

The brekkies you will find in here are just that – loaded with nutrient-dense goodness, and a little of all the macronutrients (protein, carbs and fats), to get you on track for hormonal bliss throughout your day. Oh, and they taste damn delicious! No deprivation with this way of eating!

# Coconut and Buckwheat Pancakes

Serves 2

3 eggs

3 tablespoons coconut oil, melted

¼ cup full fat coconut milk

½ teaspoon honey

¼ teaspoon organic vanilla bean powder

¼ teaspoon salt

¼ cup coconut flour

¼ cup buckwheat flour (or use all coconut flour)

1 teaspoon cinnamon powder

1 teaspoon baking soda

Extra water/coconut milk – around ½ cup

Extra coconut oil or butter, to cook

Berries, full-fat yoghurt or coconut cream, to serve

- ❧ In a bowl, whisk eggs, melted coconut oil, coconut milk and honey.
- ❧ In another bowl, mix all dry ingredients then stir in wet ingredients until smooth. You will probably need to add the extra water/coconut milk to get a pancake mix consistency – add slowly until you are satisfied with the consistency.
- ❧ Heat some coconut oil or butter in a pan over medium-high heat. Once the pan is hot, add batter (make small pancakes as they are easier to flip) and cook until brown on both sides.
- ❧ Place cooked pancakes on a plate ready to serve. (If you want to keep them warm, pop them in the oven on a low heat while you cook the rest.)
- ❧ Serve with warm berries full-fat yoghurt or coconut cream.

# Cheesy Eggs and Greens

Serves 1

1 tablespoon coconut oil
½–1 spring onion (scallion), chopped
½ medium–large zucchini, chopped
½–1 cup dark leafy greens, stems removed and chopped
A few leaves of basil (optional)
A few cherry tomatoes (optional)
Splash of apple cider vinegar
2 eggs
1 teaspoon savoury nutritional yeast flakes*
Unrefined sea salt to taste

- Melt oil over medium-high heat in a saucepan.
- Add spring onion and stir until soft.
- Add zucchini and cook until just soft.
- Turn heat to low–medium and add remaining greens (and basil and tomatoes, if using) and splash of vinegar. Cook until wilted.
- Turn heat to low and add eggs, stirring frequently to avoid eggs sticking to base.
- Once eggs are just cooked (scrambled through the greens), add yeast flakes and sea salt and stir to combine.
- Serve with avocado and/or sprouted gluten-free bread.

* Nutritional yeast, or savoury yeast flakes, are deactivated Saccharomyces cerevisiae, which is a type of yeast. They are a great vegan source of B vitamins, especially B12. Most health food stores stock this delicious 'cheesy' addition.

# Berries and Coconut Extraordinaire

Serves 1

2 handfuls mixed berries (frozen is okay; thaw what you need overnight)
1 small handful mixed nuts, chopped
Small handful pepitas and/or sunflower seeds
Small handful coconut flakes or desiccated coconut
½–1 teaspoon cinnamon
⅓ cup full-fat plain yoghurt (optional; use extra coconut milk if you wish to omit)
¼ cup full fat coconut milk
½ tablespoon melted coconut oil

❧ Stir in a bowl and enjoy!

# Banana Omelette

Serves 1

1 tablespoon coconut oil
2 eggs, whisked
½–1 teaspoon cinnamon
1 ripe banana, mashed
3 tablespoons full-fat plain yoghurt or coconut milk
1 handful of seasonal fruit
Handful nuts (optional)

❧ Heat oil in pan over medium-high heat.
❧ Mix eggs, cinnamon and banana together and pour in the pan. When browned on the outside, fold over in half as you would an omelette and cook for a little longer (but not too much, leave it moist).
❧ Serve with yoghurt or coconut milk and fruit mixed together, topped with nuts.

# Chia Pudding

Make this the night before for an easy breakfast. Let the fun begin!

Serves 2

1 cup full fat-coconut milk
3 tablespoons chia seeds
2 bananas, mashed
1–2 teaspoons cinnamon
2 small handfuls seeds (pumpkin/sunflower/flaxseed)
Coconut flakes and berries, to serve

- Mix coconut milk, chia seeds, bananas and cinnamon together in a bowl until well combined.
- Divide mix between two jars with screw top lids or two bowls.
- Allow to set in fridge overnight then top with seeds, flakes and berries in the morning.

*Note:* You can make any smoothie into a chia pudding by using the ratio of 3 tablespoons of chia seeds for every 1 cup of liquid.

# Vegetable Fritters

If you want to save time in the morning, you could mix everything together the night before then simply fry up in the morning.

Serves 1

1 cup grated sweet potato
½ medium zucchini, grated
¼ red capsicum, finely chopped
1 tablespoon shallots, chopped
4 basil leaves, chopped
½ cup leafy greens, chopped
2 eggs
1 tablespoon coconut oil
½ small avocado, sliced to serve

- ❧ Mix all ingredients, except avocado and oil, in a large bowl.
- ❧ Heat oil in pan over medium heat.
- ❧ Mould mixture into patties about 1–2 cm thick (around ½–1 cup of mix for each patty).
- ❧ Place patties in pan and allow to cook until brown on one side (approximately 5 minutes). Using a spatula, flip patties and cook for approximately 5 minutes on the other side.
- ❧ Serve with sliced avocado.

# LUNCHES AND DINNERS

For lunches and dinners, it's a good idea to mix things up throughout the week. So instead of having chicken and broccoli for dinner every night, I try to include a range of meals made from a variety of different protein sources and, of course, a load of veggies. This will ensure that you expose your guts to an abundance of vitamins, minerals, antioxidants, protein, carbs and fats. Variety is the spice of life, isn't it?

## Roast Veggie and Feta Salad

Serves 2

4 cups roast veggies such as sweet potato, beetroot, pumpkin
4 handfuls baby spinach
100 g feta, cubed (or avacado for a dairy-free option)
Small handful walnuts, chopped
Drizzle of extra virgin olive oil
Drizzle of balsamic vinegar

- ❧ Add veggies to a bowl or container.
- ❧ Top with feta and walnuts then drizzle with olive oil and balsamic vinegar.

# Asian Stir-Fry

In terms of veggies, anything goes with this meal, so feel free to ad lib. Just the other day I went shopping for this stir-fry and forgot most of the veggies. We ended up making it with just cabbage, mushrooms and red capsicum. Still worked a treat!

Serves 4–5

2 tablespoons coconut oil

1 onion, finely chopped (about ½ cup)

2 heads broccoli, sliced (about 4 cups)

2 medium carrots, sliced (about 1 cup)

500 g chicken breast or thighs, diced

2 heads baby bok choy, pak choy or silverbeet, sliced crosswise into 2-cm strips
    (about 1½ cups)

100 g mushrooms, stems removed and thinly sliced (about 1 cup)

1 small zucchini, sliced (about 1 cup)

½ teaspoon sea salt

1½ cups water

2 tablespoons arrowroot/tapioca powder, for thickening

2 tablespoons sesame oil

2 tablespoons umeboshi plum vinegar (or red wine vinegar plus extra ½ teaspoon salt)

1 tablespoon honey

- Heat the coconut oil in a large pan over medium heat.
- Sauté onion for 8–10 minutes, until soft and translucent.
- Add chicken, saute until brown.
- Add broccoli, and carrots and sauté for 10 minutes until almost tender.
- Add bok choy, mushrooms, zucchini and salt, and sauté for 5 minutes.
- Add 1 cup of the water, cover the pan, and cook for about 10 minutes, until the vegetables are wilted.

- ❧ In a small bowl, dissolve the arrowroot/tapioca powder in the remaining ½ cup of water, stirring until thoroughly combined.
- ❧ Add the arrowroot mixture to the vegetables and cook for 2–3 minutes, stirring constantly until the sauce thickens and becomes glossy.
- ❧ Stir in the sesame oil, vinegar, and honey. Serve immediately.

# Yellow Chicken Curry

Use your favourite type of chicken in this recipe; drumsticks are cheaper, but thighs are easier to cook – skin on will taste better. Use more or less curry power depending on how spicy you like it. You can also make this curry in the slow cooker. Simply throw everything in, stir and cook for 4–5 hours.

Serves 4

1 tablespoon coconut oil
1 onion, sliced
Free range chicken thighs or drumsticks (1–2 per person)
1 cup coconut cream or milk
1–2 teaspoons curry powder
Sea salt and pepper, to season

- ❧ Melt oil in frying pan over medium–high heat. Add onion and sauté until soft.
- ❧ Add chicken and brown.
- ❧ Add coconut cream/milk and curry powder and stir everything together
- ❧ Reduce heat to medium and simmer until chicken is cooked through.
- ❧ Season with salt and pepper. Serve and enjoy!

# Slow-Cooked Lamb Shanks

I find that I usually have excess sauce left over, so I blend it up and then the next day serve it with canned fish or eggs. Sounds odd, but don't knock it till you've tried it. Use homemade stock, or go for organic, without sugar or preservatives.

Serves 4

1 onion, chopped
2 celery stalks, chopped
2 carrots, peeled and chopped
3–6 garlic cloves, crushed
2 cups chicken or beef stock
1 tin no-added-salt chopped tomatoes
2 tablespoons tomato paste
1 teaspoon dried thyme (or 1–3 sprigs fresh)
2 sprigs rosemary (or 1 teaspoon dried)
1 bay leaf
4 lamb shanks
Salt and pepper, to taste
1 cup red wine

- Put the onion, celery, carrots, garlic, stock, tomatoes, tomato paste, thyme, rosemary and bay leaf in a slow cooker and stir to combine.
- Place the shanks on top of vegetables and season with salt and pepper.
- Pour in the wine, cover and cook on low for 6–10 hours. Serve, making sure to put aside 1 shank with sauce and vegetables for lunch the next day.
- Serve the sauce as is (nice and chunky), or blend everything up with a stick blender (after removing bay leaf and shanks), then pour the sauce over the shanks.

# Salmon Patties

Serves 2–3

400 g can wild-caught salmon, drained
2 eggs, beaten
¼ cup finely minced onion
1 teaspoon dried parsley
1 teaspoon mustard (sugar-free)
½ teaspoon sea salt
½ teaspoon black pepper
⅛ cup coconut/buckwheat flour
Butter/coconut oil for frying

- Place salmon in a large bowl and flake with a fork.
- Add eggs, onion, parsley, mustard, salt and pepper and stir well to mix.
- Add flour a little at a time, mixing well and stopping when the mixture will hold together in a patty shape.
- Heat some butter/coconut oil in a large frying pan over medium-high heat.
- Shape mixture into 5-cm patties; not too thick.
- Place patties into hot pan and cook until lightly brown, approximately 5–7 minutes.
- Flip the patties and cook on the other side.
- Serve with your choice of veggies.

# Ceviche

This is not in the meal plan on page 137, but I thought I would throw it in as a bonus!

### 1 Easier version

Salmon fillets (one per person), skinned, boned and cut into 1-cm cubes
Fresh lemon juice (one lemon per person)
Spring onion (½ per person), chopped
Sea salt and pepper, to taste

❧ Marinate the prepared fish in the lemon juice, spring onion and salt and pepper in a covered bowl in the fridge overnight. Serve as is.

### 2 Slightly less easy version

Serves 5–6

1 kg white firm-fleshed fish (e.g. deep sea perch, snapper) skinned, boned and cut into
   1-cm cubes
Juice of 2 lemons and 2 limes (use more, if you like)
1 Spanish onion
3 spring onions
1 red chilli, deseeded
1 small can coconut cream
1 lime, extra

❧ Marinate the prepared fish in the lemon and lime juice in a covered bowl in the fridge for at least 4 hours, or overnight.
❧ Slice Spanish onion, spring onions and deseeded red chilli and marinate for same period in the juice of 1 lime.

- After marinating, strain the fish and squeeze out any excess liquid.
- Combine with the prepared onions and chilli and add 1 small can of coconut cream.
- Season to taste with salt, pepper, and the juice of another 1–2 limes. Can be served immediately but tastes better after refrigerating for a couple of hours or the next day.

## Healthy Fish and Chips

Serves 4

¼–½ cup arrowroot/tapioca flour
¼–½ cup flat leaf parsley, chopped
4 x 150 g white fish fillets
Coconut oil or butter for frying
Sweet potato and/or parsnip, cut into fries and roasted in coconut oil and sea salt

- Mix flour and parsley together in a small bowl.
- Coat each fillet of fish in the flour/parsley mix.
- Melt oil over medium–high heat in a frying pan.
- Add fish and cook on both sides until just done (flakes away easily with a fork).
- Serve with extra veggies.

# Aaron's Marvellous Mince

My hubby Aaron is a good cook; a no-fuss cook, really. He hates reading recipes and isn't keen on spending hours in the kitchen. This mince recipe of his is a bit of a throw-together – he got lucky. Make it as is, or feel free to veer off on your own creative cooking tangent.

I find that anything mince-related tastes even better the following day. I like to up the ante and pop a poached egg on top of the leftovers for lunch. 'Cos everything is better with a poachie.

Serves 4–5

1 tablespoon coconut oil/butter
1 large onion, sliced
2 garlic cloves, chopped
500 g grass-fed beef mince
1–2 tablespoons tomato paste
1 can no-added-salt chopped tomatoes
2–3 teaspoons curry powder
1 large carrot, grated
Salt and pepper, to taste
Optional extras (choose 1, or all!):
    Mushrooms, chopped
    Kale, spinach or silverbeet, washed and chopped
    Zucchini, chopped
    Kelp, chopped

❧ Heat coconut oil/butter in pan over medium–high heat.
❧ Sauté onion and garlic until just tender.
❧ Add mince and stir until meat is slightly browned.

🌿 Add tomato paste, chopped tomatoes, curry powder and carrot and stir.

🌿 Turn heat down to low–medium and allow to simmer. Now is also the time to add in your optional extras and allow to simmer until veggies are cooked to your liking. The longer and slower this is cooked, the better it tastes. You can also make this in a slow cooker; just throw everything in, stir and cook on low for 4–6 hours.

# Snacks

Snacking is one of those controversial diet-related topics, isn't it? Should we snack? Should we not? Unfortunately, there is no hard and fast rule. If your hormones are happy, then feel free to experiment with just three meals a day (but make them decent so you're not skimping on kilojoules) for a few weeks and see how you feel. This might be good for those of you with weight-related PCOS, diabetes or obesity. If you have adrenal fatigue, hypothalamic amenorrhea, hypothyroidism, or you are pregnant or nursing, then I suggest keeping the snacks in.

When to have them? When you're hungry! Back to the whole nutrition intuition: listen to your body. If you're somewhere in-between breakfast and lunch, or lunch and dinner and you're thinking, 'Goodness gracious I'm hungry!', then go ahead and have a little snack, beautiful lady. One caveat to this: if you have one of the hormonal imbalances listed above that I recommend snacks for, you might not feel hungry (as your hormones are out of whack) and might in fact have to force yourself until things recalibrate, especially for adrenal fatigue and HA.

The snacks included here aren't your typical snacky foods that are often loaded with junk. As with the other meals, these are full of goodness that will keep your hormones happy. They're the kinds of foods you'd have in a main meal, just in smaller sizes. Enjoy!

# Fruit and Nuts

Serves 1

❧ Choose your favourite piece of fruit and team it with a handful of nuts. This will help slow down the absorption of sugars and increase the absorption of vitamins and minerals.

# Avocado and Chives

Serves 1

½ avocado
1–2 teaspoons chives, chopped
1–2 teaspoons extra virgin olive oil
1–2 teaspoons balsamic vinegar

❧ Slice avocado while still in the skin.
❧ Top with remaining ingredients and eat with a fork or spoon.

# Antipasto Skewers

Serves 1

4 olives, pitted
4 cherry tomatoes
4 cubes goat's cheese/feta (optional)
4 mini-skewers

❧ On each skewer, thread an olive, a cube of goat's cheese and a tomato. Enjoy!

# Sweet Potato Brownie

This recipe is from the fabulous George at Civilized Caveman Cooking. Check him out online; his recipes are delicious! I used 2 cups mashed orange sweet potato and I steamed the sweet potato, but you could also bake it. These brownies freeze quite well, so pack them up and save them for a rainy day (if you're able to once you taste them).

Makes 16 small serves

1 large purple sweet potato, cooked and mashed (about 2 cups)
3 eggs
¼ cup grass-fed butter, melted (or coconut oil)
¼ cup maple syrup/rice malt syrup
¼ teaspoon vanilla extract
3 tablespoons coconut flour
3 tablespoons cacao powder
2 teaspoons cinnamon
½ teaspoon ground ginger
¼ teaspoon nutmeg
¼ teaspoon baking powder
Pinch of sea salt

- Preheat oven to 175°C.
- Place sweet potato mash into a stand mixer or large mixing bowl.
- Add eggs, butter, honey and vanilla and mix well.
- Add coconut flour, cacao powder, cinnamon, ginger, nutmeg, baking powder and salt and mix until combined.
- Grease a 20-cm baking tin and pour in batter, spreading evenly.
- Place in the preheated oven and bake for 35–45 minutes or until a toothpick inserted in the centre comes out clean.
- Cool, cut, serve and enjoy.

# Anti-Inflammatory Summer Smoothie

Serves 1

½ cup full-fat coconut milk
½ cup coconut water
½ cup frozen mango
½ banana
½–1 teaspoon turmeric (start with ½ and adjust to taste; more = better for you)
½ teaspoon cinnamon
½ teaspoon ginger powder
1 teaspoon maca powder (optional)
1 tablespoon coconut oil (optional)

❧ Throw everything into a blender and whizz. Sip slowly to encourage optimal digestion.

# Green Smoothie

Serves 1

1 banana (frozen will make it creamier)
1 cup baby spinach
¼ avocado
½ teaspoon cinnamon
Sprinkle of vanilla bean powder
Coconut water or plain water to mix

❧ Blend everything together and enjoy. Sip slowly to encourage optimal digestion.

# FERMENTED FOODS

Fermented foods are essential for your daily nutritional intake and healthy hormones, not just an added bonus. Please try to get into the habit of adding 1 teaspoon (building to 1 tablespoon) of fermented veggies to each and every meal. In between meals, opt for one of the liquid ferments. You can make whey by straining a small tub of yoghurt through a muslin cloth for around 24 hours and collecting the clear liquid that strains through. What is left in the muslin cloth can be used to make homemade cream cheese – curds and whey! Little Miss Muffet was into it!

## Kate's Kombucha

Kombucha is a fermented tea. Not only is it a wonderful source of probiotics (remember I spoke about these in Chapter 4: Happy gut = happy hormones), the SCOBY converts the sugars into something called glucuronic acid, which is great for liver detoxification. SCOBY stands for symbiotic colony of bacteria and yeast – and no, it's not disgusting. You can get the kombucha mushroom from someone who has already made their own kombucha, or buy it online.

You'll need a 1-litre glass or ceramic bowl or jar and a towel/muslin cloth. Consume 100 ml per day for good health!

Makes 1 litre

1 litre filtered water
¼ cup organic sugar (to feed the SCOBY)
2 organic black tea bags
½ cup pre-made kombucha
1 SCOBY mushroom

- ❧ Sterilise the jar with boiling water and allow to air dry.
- ❧ Bring the water and sugar to a boil in a large saucepan.
- ❧ Remove from heat and pour into a glass container. I like to use a glass mixing bowl, but a wide-mouth jar does the trick too. The larger the surface area at the top, the better.
- ❧ Add tea bags, place a lid on top and allow to steep for 15 minutes.
- ❧ Remove tea bags and allow liquid to cool to around body temperature.
- ❧ Add pre-made kombucha liquid.
- ❧ Gently place SCOBY on top (it may sink to bottom; this is okay).
- ❧ Cover container with towel/cloth and secure edges. (If I use a large mixing bowl, I secure a tea towel with a few pegs; if I use a wide-mouth jar, I secure it with a rubber band or string.)
- ❧ Allow to sit for 7–10 days (7 will be plenty in warm weather). At this time you should have a baby SCOBY on top of the liquid which is very exciting. (You can use this to make other kombucha batches or give away to a friend and share the kombucha love.) The mother will be sitting at the bottom. Remove both SCOBYs and store them in a glass container with a little kombucha.
- ❧ Pour the kombucha liquid into a glass jar/bottle. Store in the fridge.

**Note:** To make it fizzy, pour kombucha into a jar with an air-tight lid, add a handful of fresh fruit (I like peaches) and screw the lid on. Let the jar sit for 2 days. Transfer to the fridge and let settle for 2 more days. Transfer to the fridge and let settle for 2 more days then BAM – you have yourself some healthy fizz!

# Sauerkraut

Makes a whole lot of kraut that will keep you going for a long time as you only need 1 teaspoon – 1 tablespoon per meal. This recipe has been adapted from **Nourishing Traditions** by Sally Fallon.

> 1 medium cabbage, cored and shredded
> 1 tablespoon caraway seeds (optional)
> 1 tablespoon sea salt
> 4 tablespoons whey (if no whey is available, add an extra tablespoon of sea salt)

- In a large bowl, mix cabbage with caraway seeds, salt and whey.
- Pound with a wooden pounder or a meat hammer or just squeeze with your hands (this is actually very soothing and meditative) for about 10 minutes to release juices.
- Place in a 1-litre wide-mouth mason jar and press down firmly with a pounder or meat hammer until juices come to the top of the cabbage. The top of the cabbage should be at least 2.5 cm below the top of the jar.
- Cover tightly and keep at room temperature for at least 7 days before transferring to the fridge.
- The sauerkraut may be eaten immediately, but it improves with age.

# Milk Kefir

Kefir is a fermented milk drink. You can use whatever milk you like for this recipe (cow, sheep, goat; whatever floats your boat). I like Nature's Goodness Kefir Turkish Yoghurt Probiotic, which you can purchase online, or at many health food stores. You can also use Body Ecology kefir grains and make according to the packet. You'll need a 1-litre mason jar, some muslin/cheesecloth and a rubber band for this recipe.

The kefir will keep for around 2 months, maybe longer. Have around ¼ cup per day to get a good dose of probiotics. I like to mix it in with my brekkie when I am having Berries and Coconut Extraordinaire (see page 216).

Makes 1 litre

1 sachet kefir or 4 tsp kefir grains
1 litre whole, unprocessed milk

❧ Pour sachet contents into jar and pour milk over the top. Stir and cover jar with cloth, securing with the rubber band.
❧ Sit on bench for 12–24 hours in warm weather (longer in cold unless you put it in front of a fan heater or next to your slow cooker). It will be ready when the top starts to get a little thicker and you see a separation of liquids. It will not be as thick as yoghurt. When you taste it, it will be tart like good quality, natural yoghurt. The longer you leave it, the more tart it will become.
❧ Remove cloth and close lid of jar. Store in fridge.

# Beet Kvass

Beet kvass is jam-packed full of nutrients and is a great digestive aid. It also helps to cleanse your liver and promote regular pooping. Good stuff!

Drink as desired. A good amount to aim for is 50–100 ml per day. You'll need a 2-litre mason jar, some muslin/cheesecloth and a rubber band. This recipe is adapted from *Nourishing Traditions* by Sally Fallon.

> 2–4 beetroots, washed and peeled (or leave skin on if organic),
>   then chopped into small cubes
> ¼ cup whey (see page 231 for recipe)
> 1 tablespoon sea salt
> Filtered water

- ❧ Place chopped beetroots in bottom of jar.
- ❧ Add whey and salt.
- ❧ Fill jar with filtered water.
- ❧ Cover with a towel or cheesecloth, secure with a rubber band and leave on the counter at room temperature for 2 days to ferment.
- ❧ Transfer to fridge.

# ORGANS AND BONES

Organs and bones are traditional super-foods and really are fundamental to a good diet and optimal hormone function. I have a friend who said he went through a stage of doing Organ Meat Sundays: he and a mate would dine on a whole bunch of nutrient-dense organ meats. On Mondays, he said, he would power through the day feeling super-human. They're that good.

## Baked Marrow Custard

This recipe is courtesy of whole-foods expert Soulla Chamberlain (go visit her awesome Broth Bar and Larder in Bronte, Sydney, Australia). It uses bone marrow. Bone marrow is an organ that is mostly made of fat. It contains unique alkylglycerols, which are special fats that boost the immune system and contain many important elements for brain growth and development.

And no, you won't taste the marrow. Instead, what you will taste is creamy deliciousness. It's a perfect dinner party dessert – they'll be none the wiser.

Serves 7

Butter or coconut oil, for greasing
50 g butter
50 g coconut oil
100 g fresh or frozen bone marrow (reserved after making bone broth)
4 eggs
200 g cream
¼ cup maple syrup
½ tablespoon vanilla bean powder
½ tablespoon cinnamon

- ❧ Preheat oven to 120°C. Grease 7 ramekins or cups with liberal amounts of butter or coconut oil.
- ❧ Melt butter, coconut oil and bone marrow in saucepan over stove very gently. Turn off heat. Add eggs, cream, maple syrup, vanilla bean powder and cinnamon and beat with a handheld blender until well mixed.
- ❧ Spoon the mixture into the ramekins, filling halfway (they will rise considerably when cooked).
- ❧ Evenly space ramekins on a baking tray and bake for 40 minutes.
- ❧ Top with whipped cream, crème fraîche, homemade vanilla ice-cream and/or a spoonful of berries if desired.

*Note:* For a dairy-free version, omit butter and substitute coconut cream for dairy cream. For a chocolate custard, add 1 cup raw cacao powder, 50g raw cacao butter and increase the sweetener (honey or maple syrup) to ¾ cup to offset the bitterness of the raw cacao powder.

# Chicken Liver Pâté

This chicken liver pâté is honestly to-die-for and is an easy way to get this super food into your diet. Try it, you won't be disappointed.

500 g organic chicken livers

6 tablespoons butter at room temperature

2 rashers bacon, chopped

1 cup chopped shallots

1 garlic clove, minced

1 large green apple, peeled, cored and chopped into cubes

1 tablespoon sage, chopped

1½ teaspoons fresh thyme leaves
¼ cup brandy
1 teaspoon sea salt
Pepper to taste
Extra butter (optional; taste as you go and add more to your liking)
Veggie sticks, to serve

- ❧ Drain the livers and set aside, giving any blood that comes off to your cat or dog. They'll love you for it, trust me. Rinse livers and allow water to drain off.
- ❧ In a large pan over medium heat, melt 2 tablespoons of butter. Add the bacon and cook, stirring occasionally, until edges are just beginning to brown.
- ❧ Add the shallots and garlic and cook, stirring occasionally, until shallots are soft.
- ❧ Add the livers, apple and herbs, and cook. Stir occasionally until the livers are just barely pink inside when cut and the apple pieces are soft.
- ❧ Transfer this mixture to your food processor.
- ❧ Pour the brandy into the pan and bring to a boil over low heat, scraping up the browned bits from the bottom of the pan.
- ❧ Boil for about 1 minute to reduce slightly, and then pour over the liver mixture.
- ❧ Add sea salt and process until mixture is very smooth, scraping down the sides of the bowl as needed.
- ❧ Transfer mixture to a bowl and mix thoroughly with the remaining 4 tablespoons of softened butter. Add pepper to taste. Pack into small jars or ramekins and smooth tops with a spatula or knife.
- ❧ Cover with extra melted butter if you are not going to gobble it all down straightaway, which I wouldn't recommend doing all by yourself.
- ❧ Refrigerate what you will eat within 3 days and freeze the rest.
- ❧ Enjoy with veggie sticks such as carrots, capsicum and cucumber.

# Bone Broth

Homemade broth/stock is a wonderfully nourishing tonic that should be enjoyed on a daily basis. A mug of warm broth is a nice way to start the day, especially in winter. You can also drink it between meals, a couple of times daily, in the afternoons when sugar cravings hit, or in the evenings after dinner. Or, if that's too far outside of your comfort zone, simply use it liberally in soups and stews.

Use bones from organic grass-fed animals; beef works best, but you can use lamb, veal or chicken. To make it really gelatinous, add some chicken feet. Sea vegetables such as kelp are optional, but provide important trace minerals such as iodine. The apple cider vinegar in this recipe is important for the extraction of minerals from the bones.

½–1 kg bones (depending on size of slow cooker/pot)
2 celery stalks, chopped
1 brown onion, chopped
6 cloves organic garlic
Sprigs of thyme, rosemary and sage
Sea vegetables such as kelp
Sea salt and pepper to taste
¼ cup apple cider vinegar
Filtered water

- Put all ingredients in slow cooker or large pot then pour in enough filtered water to cover everything.
- Set to low and let it cook for around 16 hours (6–8 hours for chicken bones).
- Allow to cool then strain broth and store in glass containers. (Mason jars work well for this.)
- In the fridge, you'll notice a layer of fat form – don't skim this off. It seals the broth and keeps it fresh. When you do break it, keep the fat to use for cooking, such as pan-frying steak.

# Goodie-Goodies

The recipes that follow are sometimes foods. They are definitely healthier than your average lolly cake (that's actually a thing here in New Zealand, cake filled with whole lollies), but they're not exactly health foods, so enjoy responsibly. And remember, **never ever** feel guilty about eating these sorts of foods. Eat them slowly and mindfully, preferably shared (everything is better when shared), and savour the whole experience.

If you're recovering from HA or an eating disorder, you might want to include these on a more regular basis. Perhaps even daily. The insulin spike you get from the natural sweetness will help with the release of GnRH (remember that one?), LH and FSH, which will help with menstruation and ovulation.

# Raw Sesame Fudge

This is a good one to enjoy if you're into seed cycling (see page 124).

Serves 3

½ cup white sesame seeds
¼ cup cacao powder
2 teaspoons raw honey (preferably Manuka)
1–2 tablespoons coconut oil
½–1 teaspoon cinnamon

- Place all ingredients in a food processor and blend well.
- Spread into a square container or on a plate and smooth the top.
- Chill in fridge (1 hour) or freezer (20 minutes) to firm. Chop and store in the freezer.

# Mum's Banana Bread

Don't you love recipes that are passed down? It's so old school! I remember coming home from school and munching down on this goodness. I hope you enjoy it as much as I did (and still do).

Makes 1 loaf

1¼ cups desiccated coconut
¼ cup coconut flour
½ cup buckwheat flour
½ cup coconut cream
1 heaped tablespoon maple syrup or rice malt syrup
2 ripe bananas, mashed
4 eggs
1 teaspoon vanilla extract
¾ teaspoon baking soda
1 teaspoon lemon juice
Butter or coconut oil, to grease

- Preheat oven to 170°C.
- Place all ingredients in food processor and blend until smooth.
- Pour into greased loaf tin (greased with butter or coconut oil, not margarine!) and leave to sit for 10 minutes.
- Bake for about 50 minutes.
- Cool before slicing. Serve as is or add a nice smear of good quality butter.

# Chocolate-Avocado Mousse

I have fooled many-a-people with this recipe. They are always completely oblivious to the fact that there is avocado in there. You can even throw in a handful of spinach if you want to be extra devious. If you don't have any avocado, you can use the flesh of one young coconut.

Serves 2–4

1 ripe avocado, mashed
½ cup cacao powder
1 teaspoon cinnamon
¼ teaspoon vanilla bean powder
1 dessertspoon raw honey
½ cup coconut water
1 tablespoon coconut oil
4 dates, finely chopped
Cream or coconut cream to serve

- Throw everything in a food processor and blend until smooth. Place mousse into a bowl, cover and refrigerate for 1–2 hours.
- Serve with fresh berries and cream/coconut cream.

# Banana Flour Carrot Muffins

This recipe is from the awesome Jo Fitton from The Primal Shift podcast. She's also a fellow member of the Ancestral Health Society of New Zealand (www.ancestralhealthnz.org), which you should definitely check out no matter where in the world you call home.

I have put it in the Goodie-Goodies section, but you could actually eat these every day – they are free of any sweetener (the carrots do that) and they are a good source of resistant starch. So go for it, they're delicious!

Makes 12 muffins

1½ cups roasted chopped carrot
½ cup oil (coconut, macadamia or ghee)
⅛ teaspoon sea salt
1 tablespoon vanilla essence
¾ cup banana flour (or buckwheat flour)
½ teaspoon baking soda
4 eggs
½ teaspoon cinnamon
½ cup liquid (water, milk, coconut milk or coconut water depending on your preference)

- ❧ Preheat oven to 180°C (160°C if fan forced).
- ❧ Mix carrots, oil, salt and vanilla in a food processer until it turns into a paste.
- ❧ Sift in banana flour and baking soda. Mix for 30 seconds.
- ❧ Add eggs and cinnamon and blend until combined.
- ❧ Mixture will be rather thick at this stage and the liquid will need to be added until mixture has the consistency of a thick batter.
- ❧ Pour into a lined muffin tray and bake for 15–20 minutes. Keep checking the muffins as they are cooking because they can dry out quickly.

# Lemon Gelatin Mousse

Not only is gelatin super-nourishing for your gut but wonderful for encouraging luscious locks, glowing skin and strong nails. On top of this, gelatin-rich foods help nourish your joints and improves digestion. I like Great Lakes brand gelatin powder; Sarah Wilson from I Quit Sugar has a good one too.

Serves 4

1 cup full-fat coconut milk
Juice from 1–2 lemons (depending on how lemony you like it)
Rind from ¾ of a lemon
1–2 tablespoons honey (depending on how sweet you like it)
¼–½ teaspoon vanilla bean powder or 1 teaspoon vanilla extract
1 tablespoon gelatin powder
2 tablespoons water
Fresh berries and/or coconut flakes, to serve

- Place coconut milk, lemon juice, lemon rind, honey and vanilla in a saucepan over medium heat and whisk.
- Combine gelatin and water in a small bowl.
- Add gelatin mix to the saucepan and stir well until dissolved.
- When the mixture is warm, transfer into 2–4 small serving dishes (e.g. ramekins or cups).
- Place in the fridge for 30-45 minutes (or freezer to set faster).
- Serve as is or with fresh berries and/or coconut flakes.

# Baked Berry Custard

Serves 2

1 cup full-fat coconut milk (or your milk of choice)

3 eggs

⅓ teaspoon vanilla powder

1 tablespoon maple syrup (not maple-flavoured syrup)

2 tablespoons coconut oil, melted

½–1 teaspoon cinnamon

Handful of berries (I like blueberries, but any will work)

Sprinkle of nutmeg (optional)

- Preheat oven to 160°C.
- Blend all ingredients other than berries and nutmeg (I use a stick/immersion blender).
- Divide berries between 2 ramekins and pour mix over the top.
- Sprinkle with a little nutmeg, if desired.
- Bake for 45 minutes.

# NOT THE END,
# BUT THE BEGINNING

Now we've come to the end of the book, but it should be just the beginning of your health and wellness journey. I truly hope that the strategies in this book not only help happify your hormones and help you live a long, healthy and vibrant life, but also that you now have a sense of, 'Ahhh, so that's what's going on in my body. Now I know what I need to do and why I need to do it.' Empowerment and all that, you know?

So, my beautiful ladies, I thank you for reading this book, and putting up with my extensive waffle. Finally, I leave you with this dedication...

*Namaste*

*My soul honours your soul.*

*I honour the place in you where the entire universe resides.*

*I honour the light, love, truth, beauty and peace within you,*

*because it is also within me.*

*In sharing these things we are united, we are the same.*

*We are one.*

*Be kind to yourself, gorgeous.*

*Much love,*

*Kate xx*

# GREAT COOKBOOKS

If you're hankering for some more food porn, here are a few of my favourite real-food cookbooks.

*Nourishing Traditions*, Fallon, Sally et al., NewTrends Publishing, 2001.

*Heal Your Gut*, Holmes, Lee, Murdoch Books, Sydney, 2015.

*I Am Food*, Koullouros, Anthia, Penguin Publishing, Sydney, 2014.

*Eat Drink Paleo*, Macri, Irena, Michael Joseph, London, 2015.

*The Unbakery: Raw Organic Goodness*, May, Megan, Beatnik Publishing, New Zealand, 2014.

*Practical Paleo*, Sanfilippo, Diane, Victory Belt Publishing, USA, 2012.

*Dr Libby's Real Food Chef*, Weaver, Libby, and Cynthia Louise, Little Green Frog Publishing, New Zealand, 2013.

*Dr Libby's Real Food Kitchen*, Weaver, Libby, and Cynthia Louise, Little Green Frog Publishing, New Zealand, 2013.

*I Quit Sugar – Simplicious*, Wilson, Sarah, Pan Macmillan Australia Pty Ltd, Australia, 2015.

*Optimum Health the Paleo Way*, Yates, Claire, Exisle Publishing, Wollombi, 2013.

# ACKNOWLEDGEMENTS

Thank you to Sam at Finch Publishing for kindly offering me the opportunity to write this book. It was something I have always wanted to do, but needed a little external kick in the bum to do so. Thank you also to Jenny, my editor, for sorting through my waffle, reining me in, and making this thing legible.

Oodles of gratitude to my amazing husband, who has always supported me in every way possible. Thank you, especially, for being such an awesome father to our Little O. Without you, none of this would be possible.

Thank you to my daughter, Olivia, for making me laugh and providing inspiration to share this message with other women so that hopefully the younger generation grow up to be kinder to themselves than we have been to ourselves.

I am grateful to my parents, for always encouraging me to follow my heart and do what it so desires.

Thank you to those who contributed recipes: Soulla Chamberlain, Jo Fitton, George Bryant, Az (hubby), and Mum. (Though I don't think she knew she was contributing. Oops! Thanks, Mum!)

Last but certainly not least, I am grateful to all of the women out there (and men; there are a handful of you, I know) who have been so incredibly supportive of me through my own hormonal woes, and for helping me to spread this important message. So much love to you all.

Kate xx

# END NOTES

p17 'When Dr Price analysed the foods used by isolated primitive peoples, he found that in comparison to the American diet of his day they provided at least four times the calcium and other minerals.' Weston A Price 2000, 'Weston A Price – DDS', accessed 28 Feb 2016, www.westonaprice.org/health-topics/weston-a-price-dds/.

p17 'If you're interested in learning more about Dr Price's research, I can highly recommend his book, *Nutrition and Physical Degeneration*.' Weston A. Price, *Nutrition and Physical Degeneration*, Price-Pottenger Nutrition Foundation, USA, 2008.

p64 'A microbiome is the ecological community of commensal, symbiotic and pathogenic microorganisms that literally share our body space.' National Institute of Health 2016, 'Human Microbiome Project DACC', accessed 28 Feb 2016, hmpdacc.org.

p75 'Time to become a poop detective! Sounds fun, right? Have you ever heard of the Bristol Stool Chart?' SJ Lewis & KW Heaton, 'Stool form scale as a useful guide to intestinal transit time', *Scandinavian Journal of Gastroenterology*, Vol 32, no. 9, 1997, pp. 920–4.

p98 Use the 'Dirty Dozen and Clean Fifteen' list from the Environmental Working Group to help you decide which veggies are best to buy organic.' Environmental Working Group 2016, 'Consumer Guides', accessed 29 Feb 2016, www.ewg.org/consumer-guides.

p101 'Preparing grains properly' Thanks to *Nourishing Traditions*, by Sally Fallon for providing such an awesome resource on preparation of whole foods to maximise nutrition and minimise any adverse effects! S Fallon et al., *Nourishing Traditions*, NewTrends Publishing, USA, 2001.

p101 'Many brain disorders have been implicated with gluten consumption, including schizophrenia and autism.' Whitely, P., Rodgers. J., Savery, D., Shattock, P., 'A gluten-free diet as an intervention for autism and associated spectrum disorders: preliminary findings' published in *Autism*, Sage Publications and The National Autistic Society, Vol 3(1) 45–65; 007675 1362-3613(199903)3:1, 1999. 'Markers of Celiac Disease and Gluten Sensitivity in Children with Autism', Lau M. N, Green, H., Taylor, K., et al in *PLOS One* Journal, June 18, 2013. Kalaydjian A.E., Eaton W., Cascella N., Fasano A., 'The gluten connection: the association between schizophrenia and celiac disease.' PUB Med.gov, 2006 Feb;113(2):82-90.<see http://www.ncbi.nlm.nih.gov/pubmed/16423158. Karolinska Institutet. 'Maternal gluten sensitivity linked to schizophrenia risk in children.' ScienceDaily. www.sciencedaily.com/releases/2012/05/120511101242.htm (accessed June 22, 2016).

p101 'And did you know that non-coeliac gluten sensitivity is a real thing? Smart science peeps have been studying it for a while.' Holmes, G., 'Non-coeliac gluten sensitivity', Royal Derby Hospital, Derby, UK Gastroenterol Hepatol Bed Bench 2013;6(3):115-119

p103 'See more about this on my blog and in my e-book *Healing Hypothalamic Amenorrhea*.' K Callaghan, *Healing Hypothalamic Amenorrhea: An Ancestral Guide to a Modern Girl's Dilemma*, 1st ed, www.theholisticnutritionist.com/ebook, Kate Callaghan, New Zealand, 2015.

p104 'It's pretty simple to get a rough estimate of how many kilojoules you need on a daily basis. Just plug your own personal values into the appropriate equation.' WN Schofield, 'Predicting basal metabolic rate: new standards and review of previous work', *Human Nutrition – Clinical Nutrition*, vol 39 Suppl, 1985, pp. 5-41.

p147 'Menopause is pretty much the only conditionI recommend soy for. Otherwise I say there is no joy in soy!' K Daniel, *The Whole Soy Story*, NewTrends Publishing, USA, 2005.

p165 'In one study a small number of women were treated with hypothalamic amenorrhea with leptin over a period of three months and found that the treatment did restore menstruation, ovulation and hence, fertility.' CK Welt et al, 'Recombinant Human Leptin in Women with Hypothalamic Amenorrhea', *Obstetrical & Gynecological Survey*, vol 60.2, 2005, pp. 104–105.

p165 'In another study, leptin therapy resulted in 70 per cent of women getting their period back, and 60 per cent of these women also ovulated.' CS Mantzoros et al, 'Leptin in Human Physiology and Pathophysiology', *The American Journal of Physiology – Endocrinology and Metabolism*, vol 301, 2011, pp. E567-E584.

p167 'My favourite online yoga resource, for those of you who can't make it to classes, is YogaGlo.' YogaGlo, Inc. 2016, 'Yogaglo', accessed 28 Feb. 2016, http://www.yogaglo.com.

p203 'I can highly recommend checking out the work of Louise Hay.' L Hay, *You Can Heal Your Life*, Hay House, Santa Monica, 1987.

p203 'I can highly recommend checking out the work of Gabrielle Bernstein.' G Bernstein, *May Cause Miracles*, Hay House, London, 2013.

p207 'Self-criticism is not 'love', and it is certainly not indifferent. It's a form of hatred.' D LaPorte, Danielle 2010, 'Self Hatred: Beneath Sugar-Coated Criticism', accessed 29 Feb 2016, www.daniellelaporte.com/self-hatred-beneath-sugar-coated-criticism/.

p229 'This recipe is from the fabulous George at Civilized Caveman Cooking.' G Bryant, 'Paleo Recipes – Civilized Caveman®', *Civilized Caveman Cooking Creations*, accessed 29 Feb 2016, http://www.civilizedcavemancooking.com.

p233 'Sauerkraut recipe adapted from *Nourishing Traditions* by Sally Fallon.' S Fallon et al., *Nourishing Traditions*, NewTrends Publishing, USA, 2001.

p235 'Beet kvass recipe adapted from *Nourishing Traditions* by Sally Fallon.' S Fallon et al., *Nourishing Traditions*, NewTrends Publishing, USA, 2001.

p236 'This recipe is courtesy of whole-foods expert Soulla Chamberlain (go visit her awesome Broth Bar and Larder in Bronte, Sydney, Australia).' Star Anise Organic Wholefoods 2016, 'Traditional Wholefoods for a Modern World', accessed 20 Feb 2016, http://www.staraniseorganic.com.

p243 'This recipe is from the awesome Jo Fitton from The Primal Shift podcast.' J Fitton 2016, 'The Primal Shift, Practical Approaches for Primal Living in a Modern World', accessed 29 Feb 2016, www.theprimalshift.com.au.

Printed in Australia
AUHW011013160123
373298AU00004B/4